Natural Healing Foods

A User Friendly Reference to Nature's Pharmacy

Natural Healing Foods

A User Friendly Reference to Nature's Pharmacy

By Pamela Young

Natural Healing Foods
©Pamela Young, 2011. All rights reserved. No part of this publication may be reproduced, stored in a retrieval system, or transmitted in any form or by any means, electronic, mechanical photocopying, recording, scanning, or otherwise, except as permitted under Section 107 or 108 of the 1976 United States Copyright Act, without the prior written permission of the publisher.

ISBN 978-0-9840804-2-7

Library of Congress Control Number: 2010938876

First Edition Published August 1, 2011.

Printed in the USA using CPSIA compliant materials.

∞ This paper meets the requirements of ANSI/NISO Z39.48-1992 (Permanence of Paper)

Cover Image © Mikie11, 2011. All images used under license from Shutterstock.com.
Book and cover design by Darlene Swanson of Van-garde Imagery, Inc.

CAVU Publishing
Scottsdale, Arizona

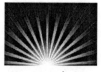

www.cavupubs.com

For my mother, Ruby, who at 90 is an inspiration to everyone she meets.

Contents

Part II – Helpful Herbs and Spices

Part III– Health Problems

Preface

If you're like most people, you try to do your best to stay as healthy as you can. You visit your doctor for annual tests to monitor your health, and work with your physician to maintain or regain good health.

Your doctor, being the careful physician he or she is, remarks your cholesterol level is elevated. He recounts the dangers of heart disease and suggests you exercise more and cut out pies and desserts on a daily basis. He recommends beginning a daily regimen of a cholesterol reducing drug.

At first you resist the idea of pills, thinking you will certainly do better with your diet and exercise. For the next week or so you do a stellar job watching what you eat and hopping on the treadmill daily, but soon life intervenes. There's just not enough time for the gym, and with everything else happening in your life, fast food is the easiest and quickest solution for lunch - and often dinner.

A few weeks later, it's back to the doctor for your follow-up appointment and the test results are grim. Your bad cholesterol level is creeping higher and, with the stern warning from your doctor your health is in danger, you reluctantly give in and accept the drugged route to health. The price tag tops at $150 a month. (Remember when you thought $50 for vitamins was insane?) But, unfortunately, there's no hard evidence guaranteeing the drug will prolong your life, or even improve its quality, especially when you consider side effects of the drug include strokes, or even death.

Welcome to reality - you are now caught in the web of big pharmaceutical companies slowly transferring *your* wealth to their bottom line profits, and it's for the rest of your life.

The really sad part of this story is simply this - it is all unnecessary. Heart disease is the number one cause of death in the United States today for both men and women. Cancer is number two. Did you know 150 years ago heart disease was virtually unknown? In 1850 the leading causes of death were pneumonia, influenza, tuberculosis, diarrhea, and infection. Cancer in the year 1850 affected only three in 100 people. Today that number has exploded to 28 in 100 people, and the number is rising each year. Why the change? It's due to many reasons, but before we explore them, let's travel back in time.

In the Beginning

Before physicians, hospitals, and pharmaceutical companies existed, there were "healers," people who lived close to the land and discovered natural cures for illness. Healers were mostly women because they were the gatherers and nurturers. Their "cures" utilized natural foods such as vegetables, fruits, seeds, nuts, grains, and herbs. Their wisdom was passed down through the ages from one generation to the next.

Fast forward to ancient Greece and the time in history when healing was turned over to the men. Hippocrates (ca. 460 BC – 370 BC) is known as the father of Western medicine. His father, Heraclites, was also a physician, but Hippocrates rejected the then current belief that all illness came as a punishment from the gods. Instead, he felt man caused his own problems – not the gods. Because of his sacrilege, Hippocrates was imprisoned for twenty years. During those years of confinement, he continued to study medicine. He determined since all illness had a natural cause, then it must also have a natural cure.

Hippocrates defined disease as "suffering and strain," and proposed nutrition was the key to good health. "Thy food shall by thy medicine," he said. "Thy medicine shall by thy food." The father of Western medicine recognized there was a natural balance in all things and the human body was no exception. He called this balance "homeostasis," which Eastern medicine defines as Yin and Yang. Hippocrates felt when the body is out of balance, nutritionally or emotionally, it becomes more susceptible to illness. He also felt the human body was remarkable with its self-healing abilities.

Hippocrates proposed, "If we could give every individual the right amount of nourishment and exercise, not too little and not too much, we would have found the safest way to health."

Two-time Nobel Prize winner Dr. Linus Pauling (1901 – 1994) also found disfavor in the scientific community for his theories on nutrition - specifically vitamin therapy. He wrote "Vitamin C and the Common Cold" in 1970, which emphatically stated large doses of vitamin C could combat flu, infections, cancer, heart disease and even old age. He further stated vitamins like B and E worked to fight disease and prolong life.

Although scientists fought hard to disprove his theories by conducting their own research, Dr. Pauling found many of their studies were flawed. He often proved them wrong with his own research and logical reasoning. Pauling died of cancer at the age of 93, but said vitamin C delayed the cancer's onset for twenty years.

Prolific inventor and genius Thomas Edison (1847 – 1931) also strongly advocated nutritional medicine. He noted, "The doctor of the future will give no medicine, but will interest his patients in the care of the human frame, in diet, and the cause and prevention of disease."

Today We Are in a Mine Field in Our Quest for Good Health

There have been great strides in the field of medicine in the 21st century. Wonder drugs have been purported to relieve the symptoms of many illnesses, thus most doctors today have distanced themselves from the concept of natural healing through nutrition. Instead, medical schools focus on pharmacology, anatomy, biochemistry, physiology, microbiology, pathology, medical ethics, and laws governing medicine. Very little importance or credence is given to diet. At Harvard Medical School, less than two percent of a student's time is spent studying preventative medicine, and only a small portion of that time is spent studying nutrition. Instead, primary emphasis is focused on pharmacology. This approach seems to take a defensive reaction once a disease is diagnosed, utilizing drug therapy rather than proactively preventing the disease in the first place – much to the appreciation of drug companies.

According to Fortune Magazine's Global 500 report in 2009, the top ten pharmaceutical companies had combined revenues of $393 billion dollars. It's an eye-watering number, especially when you consider there are thousands of drug companies busily lobbying our doctors to prescribe their drugs. Worse, the pharmaceutical companies advertise in magazines and on television encouraging people to ask their doctors to prescribe their drugs. It's a never ending cycle, and our dependence on manufactured drugs is to their good fortune.

Unfortunately, many drugs cause unwanted side effects including other illnesses, toxicity, and even death. Dr. Julian Whitacker, a graduate of Dartmouth College and Emory University Medical School, recently said, "Millions of Americans swallow pills that are supposed to make them feel better — physically or mentally — but covertly wreak havoc with their bodies and brains. Many older folks are diagnosed as senile, when in fact their drugs are causing their memory lapses and confusion."

Not only are we becoming addicted to drugs, but we're also becoming obese. Diabetes is at an all time high. Why is this happening?

The second land mine we encounter relates to how our food is being raised and produced these days. In the United States today, approximately 36 million cattle are raised to provide beef for American consumers. In the interest of capitalism, two thirds (about 24 million cows) are given steroids and hormones to speed growth and produce bigger, fatter cows. The same process is used for poultry.

As we consume beef, chicken, eggs, and even cow's milk, we are ingesting steroids and hormones into our own bodies. These steroids and hormones have been linked to weight gain, diabetes, and even cancer. Just as farmers are using drugs to raise their animals faster, food producers are using chemicals to grow, process and preserve the food we eat. In fact, over 14,000 man-made chemicals are added to the foods we consume today. Although too many to discuss here, the common culprits are artificial sweeteners (Acesulfame K) known to cause cancer in animals; artificial colorings, again a carcinogen; BHA and BHT, chemicals to prevent oxidation and retard rancidity, also highly suspect carcinogens, and finally nitrites and nitrates which are meat preservatives, suspected of causing stomach cancer.

Olestra, a fake fat, has also been linked to cancer. The Harvard

School of Public Health stated, ". . . the long term consumption of oles-tra snack foods might therefore result in several thousand unnecessary deaths each year from lung and prostate cancers and heart disease, and hundreds of additional cases of blindness in the elderly due to macular degeneration."

Sodium bromate, used to increase the volume of bread, is a suspected carcinogen which has been banned in most of the world–except in the United States and Japan. Sulfites, used to keep fruits and vegetables looking fresh, can cause severe allergic reactions. Carboxymethylcellu-lose, a stabilizer used in ice cream, salad dressing, cheese spreads, and chocolate milk is a highly suspected carcinogen. In laboratory experi-ments this stabilizer has resulted in cancer in 80 percent of rats tested.

We are also exposed to metals in food production processes that could have fatal results. Aluminum, found in baking powder, beer, bake ware, cosmetics, toothpaste, antiperspirants, aspirin and even tap wa-ter, has been linked to Alzheimer's disease, Parkinson's disease, kidney dysfunction, and ulcers. Arsenic, used in pesticides, insect sprays and found in seafood from coastal waters, has been linked to skin cancer, anemia, and esophageal problems. Cadmium, found in candy, coffee, soft drinks, and batteries, has been linked to cancer, cerebral hemor-rhage, and liver damage. Copper, found in birth control pills, beer, cookware, corn oil, lobster, and avocados, has been linked to Hodgkin's disease, cancer, autism, multiple sclerosis, high blood pressure, dia-betes, and schizophrenia. Lead, found in canned fruit juices, hair dye, toothpaste, milk, and toys, has been linked to arthritis and joint pain, Parkinson's disease, multiple sclerosis, and renal dysfunction. Mer-cury, found in fish, cereals, hemorrhoid products, dental amalgams, soft contact lens solutions, and certain medications, has been linked to adrenal dysfunction, deafness, schizophrenia, and vision loss.

Additionally, pesticides have been linked to sterility and cancer. In 1977, workers at a pesticide plant in California discovered they had been rendered sterile due to exposure of DBCP, (1,2-Dibromo-3-chloropropane). Although most companies suspended production because of its "carcinogenic and mutagenic" properties, one company did not. Company management stated, "It was our opinion that a vacuum existed in the marketplace that (we) could temporarily occupy... (and) with the addition of DBCP, sales might be sufficient to reach a profitable level." The Environmental Protection Agency investigated the chemical and after two years, banned it in the U.S.

Unfortunately, that's not the end of the story. DBCP, although banned in the U.S., is currently being exported to foreign countries where it is sprayed on bananas and then that fruit is shipped back into the U.S. for consumption. The fact is, imported produce is more likely to be highly poisonous than produce grown in America. Why? As a Mexican agribusinessman said recently, "Americans eat with their eyes. They won't buy a fruit or vegetable with any insect marks or blemishes, so we spray them heavily. About four times as much spray as we use on our own domestic crops. No insects ever touch that food."

So What Can You Do?

First, realize you have more power than you think. You can avoid all the land mines adversely affecting your body simply by being more proactive with your health. Learn to read labels on packaged foods. If you don't understand an ingredient (or can't pronounce it) chances are it's not good for you. Concentrate your shopping on the most natural foods you can find. Many grocery stores are now adding organic fruits and vegetables to their produce departments. Throughout the world there are farmer's markets, often with stands featuring locally grown, organic produce. Try to buy foods from the source as much as possible. When you do shop in markets, buy beef and chicken from stores labeling their meat as hormone free—and that includes eggs and milk.

Your second line of defense in your quest for good health is to arm yourself with knowledge. The key to optimum health is to not only add nutritious foods into our bodies, but to eliminate toxins. The best and easiest way to eliminate toxins is to add fiber to your diet. Whole wheat flour instead of white flour is best. Brown rice, with the nutritional hull, is better than white rice. Beans are extremely high in fiber, as are fruits and vegetables. Nuts and seeds are also a good source of fiber. To make it easy, the fiber content of each of the foods mentioned in this book is listed.

Realize, too, herbs are another important way to eliminate toxins. The healers of the past knew the value of dandelion as a purifier of your system. Did you ever hear of "spring tonic?" Way back when, that tonic was comprised of dandelion greens. Both dandelion and red clovers purify our blood and eliminate toxins.

Vitamins also play an important role in preventing illness. Most vitamins we need are naturally found in the foods we eat, but supplements are helpful since there are times when we don't always eat properly.

You have probably heard stress is a killer, but do you know why? Stress depletes the body of vitamins, specifically vitamin B. Without a balance of vitamins in our bodies, our immune system is compromised and we become vulnerable to disease. It's important to keep vitamins A, B, C, D and E well-balanced in our bodies.

As important as it is to eat the correct foods, it's equally important to avoid bad foods. Sugar, unfortunately, is not good for our systems. It causes irritation and weakening of the mucous membranes in our bodies and robs teeth and blood of minerals. Sugar can actually leach vitamins B, C and D as well as calcium, iron and zinc from our bodies, leading to osteoporosis. Carbonated beverages are not good for you. They leach calcium from our bones, as well as adding caffeine, which has been linked to high blood pressure and heart disease.

Red meat is another food that can cause health problems. Red meat, because of its high fat content, not only raises cholesterol levels, but has been associated with heart disease, colon cancer, arthritis, joint pain, and diabetes. Salt is yet another culprit harmful to our health. Too much salt can cause elevated blood pressure, asthma, osteoporosis and even stroke.

Fish is an excellent source of protein, and it's a good choice to make in the quest for good health. However, recently there have been concerns raised about the safety of fish due to high levels of mercury and other contaminants. To help clarify which fish to buy, the Monterey Bay Aquarium released their "Super Green" list of seafood. Some of their suggestions include:

- Albacore Tuna (troll or pole caught in U.S/British Columbia)

- Salmon (wild, caught in Alaska)

- Oysters (farmed)

- Rainbow Trout (farmed)

- Arctic Char (farmed)

- Barramundi (farmed in the U.S.)

- Longfin Squid (wild-caught in the Atlantic)

- Mussels (farmed)

- Pink Shrimp (wild caught in Oregon)

- Spot Prawns (wild caught in British Columbia)

- Pacific Sardines (wild caught)

What Led Me to Write Natural Healing

Natural Healing Foods verifies, with extensive clinical research, that old ways work. Not only do they work as well as drugs in many cases, but unlike drugs, there are little to no side effects.

The research for this book began 25 years ago. At that time I was working in a job requiring me to carry an extremely heavy briefcase. I ended up with carpal tunnel in my right arm. Unable to pick up something as light as a plate, I immediately contacted my doctor who told me the inflammation in my arm was so intense I needed to immobilize my arm immediately to prevent further damage. So he encased my arm in a cast. The cast was to be worn for several weeks, and if the inflammation persisted, surgery would be in order.

Unfortunately, within a week my arm began to swell inside the cast. The doctor wanted to replace it with another one. In the process of removing the old cast, he sliced my arm with the saw. By this time I was beginning to get a bad feeling about having another cast put on, so I told him not to do it. He said if I didn't wear a cast to keep my arm rigid, at the very least I would have to go through weeks of physical therapy with the possibility of surgery still in my future.

I certainly didn't want to jeopardize my health by being stubborn, but somewhere deep inside I knew there had to be a better way. After I left my doctor's office, I remembered an article I read some time before about herbs helping people suffering from inflammation.

I headed to the library and looked through all the books I could find about herbs and their healing properties. The one herb mentioned again and again to fight inflammation was yucca. My next stop was the health food store. Knowing nothing about herbs, I asked the gentleman manning the store if he carried yucca. He immediately went to a shelf and picked up a small bottle containing 100 capsules.

I shared I had never taken herbs before and was a bit nervous about the whole thing. He explained herbs were different from pharmaceutical drugs in that drugs were meant to relieve symptoms immediately, but herbs took longer to take effect. He instructed me to follow the directions on the bottle, and assured me I should notice results in a few weeks.

Not knowing how my body was going to react to yucca, I only took half the dose per day. Within two weeks I not only could lift plates, but bowling balls! I was delighted I avoided surgery, but even more, I was amazed at the immense healing power of herbs.

The most important revelation of that whole experience was we all have the power to heal ourselves. It was as if a light finally turned on. If yucca could help heal carpal tunnel syndrome, what other diseases could be helped by herbs? As I began to do more and more research, I discovered not only herbs, but foods and even spices were powerful tools to keep us healthy.

Twenty-five years ago, doctors often referred to the healing power of food and herbs as "folklore and quackery," but through the years, increasing numbers of doctors and hospitals—including the famous Mayo Clinic—are beginning to realize the healing connection between nutrition and disease. Although I am not a doctor, I am an avid health researcher and I firmly believe nature has provided a cure for every disease known to man. I also believe scientists will eventually discover and medically accept plants or foods that truly do help us heal.

In 2010 as I was researching this book, my mother who was 89 at the time, began to suffer digestive problems. She no longer cared about food and began to lose weight. I told her she needed to check with her doctor to find out what was wrong. Her doctor told her she had gall stones and would probably need surgery. Unfortunately, the operation could not be scheduled for two weeks. I was concerned because she was so uncomfortable.

While researching for this book, I found apple cider vinegar is an effective flush for gallstones, and I asked my mother what she thought about it. She remembered as a child, her mother told her about the curative powers of apple cider vinegar and agreed to give it a try. She began by mixing two tablespoons of apple cider vinegar with two tablespoons of honey in an eight-ounce glass of water and drinking it twice a day. Within a week she was feeling better and her appetite improved. When she next saw her doctor, he confirmed she no longer had the problem and did not need an operation. Today, at almost 90, she's doing great and has not had a recurrence of gall stones.

There are many books on the subject of food and healing, but I have found them to be cumbersome to read – especially when you want an answer immediately. Because of this, I have intentionally made *Natural Healing Foods* as "user-friendly" as possible so when information is needed, answers are quickly found. The first section of the book is an alphabetical listing titled Foods; the second section covers Herbs and Spices, and the last section addresses Diseases – an easy reference without having to wade through paragraph after paragraph for answers.

I leave you with one thought. For many years, the United States has been recognized for its excellent health care system. However, with the recently passed health care law, Americans may be facing limited health care choices, overcrowded conditions, and a bureaucratic maze to navigate just to receive the simplest treatments. Health care may be available for all, but with more patients and fewer doctors to provide services, the quality of health care may not be what we have experienced in the past. It is now up to all of us to work on taking charge of our own health *before* we have a problem. Nutrition is the first step. Being proactive about your health and staying healthy is far better than being reactive and trying to cure a disease once it has taken hold. Remember, we are the choices we make. If we don't take care of our own health, someone will take care of it for us. Don't give that power to another person!

Good health to you!

Organic and Non-Organic Foods

The Environmental Working Group (an organization of scientists, researchers and policymakers) has composed a list of produce you should always buy in organic form. Even after a thorough washing, these fruits and vegetables still tested positive for between 47 and 67 different chemicals.

Fruits & Vegetables Best Bought in Organic Form Include:

Apples

Blueberries

Carrots

Celery

Cherries

Collard Greens

Grapes (Imported)

Kale

Lettuce

Nectarines

Peaches

Pears

Peppers (Sweet)

Potatoes

Raspberries

Spinach

Strawberries

Fruits And Vegetables That Are Safe To Buy Non-Organic Include:

Asparagus

Avocados

Cabbage

Mango

Cantaloupe

Onions

Corn

Peas

Eggplant

Pineapples

Grapefruit

Sweet Potatoes

Kiwi

Watermelon

Part I

The Healing Foods

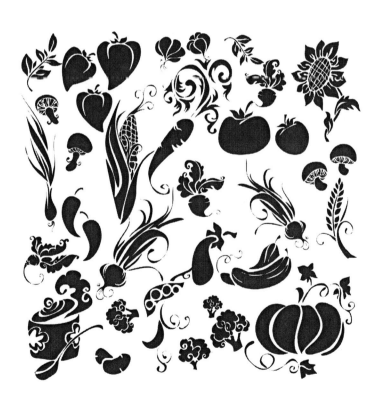

Almonds

According to a study done by David Jenkins M.D., PhD, D.Sc., Department of Sciences at the University of Toronto, individuals who ate a handful of almonds every day lowered their bad cholesterol level by 4.4%, and those who ate two handfuls of almonds every day lowered their bad cholesterol by 9.4%.

Aging
Alzheimer's Disease
Anemia
Arthritis/Joint Pain
Atherosclerosis
Blood Pressure
Bursitis
Cancer
Cholesterol
Circulation
Colon
Constipation
Cramps
Depression
Diabetes
Diverticulitis
Energy
Eyes
Fibromyalgia

Fingernails/Hair
Gall Stones
Gout
Heart Disease
Hemorrhoids
Immune System
Inflammation
Liver
Lungs
Multiple Sclerosis
Muscles/Ligaments
Obesity
Osteoporosis
Premenstrual Syndrome
Skin
Stress
Stroke
Thyroid/Goiter
Ulcers

One ounce (23 whole almonds) has 161 calories,
14 grams fat (1g saturated), 3 grams fiber, 16 grams carbohydrates.

*"Leave your drugs in the chemist's pot
if you can heal the patient with food."*

—Hippocrates

Apple Cider Vinegar

A 2005 study at Arizona State University revealed that apple cider vinegar slowed the increase of blood sugar when consumed before high-carbohydrate meals, important in preventing type 2 diabetes.

Acne	Gout
Aging	Headache
Allergies	Heartburn
Arthritis/Joint Pain	Hemorrhages
Asthma	Hemorrhoids
Blood Pressure	Influenza
Cancer	Insomnia
Cholesterol	Kidneys
Colds	Nervousness
Colitis	Obesity
Constipation	Phlegm
Cramps	Premenstrual Syndrome
Diabetes	Rheumatism
Diarrhea	Shingles
Energy	Sinus
Eyes	Skin
Fatigue	Teeth/Gums
Fibromyalgia	Ulcers
Fingernails/Hair	Varicose Veins
Gall Stones	

One tablespoon of apple cider vinegar has no calories,
no fat, no fiber, and no carbohydrates.

"An apple a day keeps the doctor away."

—Your mother

Apples

An apple a day can help keep breast cancer away, according to a lab study by food scientists at Cornell University. "We found that tumor incidence was reduced by 17, 39 and 44 percent in animals fed the human equivalent of one, three or six apples a day, respectively, over 24 weeks," says Rui Hai Liu, Cornell associate professor of food science and lead author of the study.

Acne

Allergies

Alzheimer's Disease

Anemia

Arthritis/Joint Pain

Asthma

Blood Pressure

Breast Cancer

Bronchitis

Cancer

Cervical Cancer

Cholesterol

Circulation

Colds

Colon

Colon Cancer

Constipation

Cramps

Diabetes

Diarrhea (applesauce)

Digestion

Diverticulitis

Energy

Eyes

Fibromyalgia

Gall Stones (apple juice)

Gallbladder

Gout

Heart Disease

Heartburn

Hemorrhoids

Hepatitis

Immune System

Inflammation

Influenza

Irritable Bowel Syndrome

Kidneys

Liver

Lungs

Menopause

Multiple Sclerosis

Muscles/Ligaments

Nausea (apple juice)

Nervousness

Obesity

Osteoporosis

Pain

Parkinson's Disease

Pneumonia

Prostate

Radiation exposure

Rheumatism

Rosacea

Shingles

Sinus

Stomach Cancer

Stroke

Teeth/Gums

Ulcerative Colitis

Ulcers

Varicose Veins

One medium apple has 71 calories,
no fat, 3 grams fiber,19 grams carbohydrates

Apricots

Hard as it is to believe, some people claim apricots are the secret to living to age 120. The Hunzas, a tribe living in the Himalayan Mountains of Asia are some of the longest living people on earth. Common health problems, like cancer, heart disease, high blood pressure, and high cholesterol, do not exist in the Hunza. And researchers are wondering if apricots, a main part of their diet, are partly responsible. The Hunzas eat fresh apricots in season and dry the rest to eat during their long, cold winter.

Aging
Alzheimer's Disease
Anemia
Blood Pressure
Cancer
Circulation
Colon
Constipation
Cramps
Digestion
Diverticulitis
Emphysema
Eyes
Gall Stones
Gallbladder
Heart Disease

Hemorrhoids
Inflammation
Irritable Bowel Syndrome
Lupus
Multiple Sclerosis
Nausea (canned
    apricots are best)
Obesity
Pain
Prostate
Rosacea
Shingles
Sinus
Skin
Stress
Stroke
Urinary Tract

One medium apricot has 16 calories, no fat,
1 gram fiber, 4 grams carbohydrates.

Artichokes

The artichoke has been used for liver and gallbladder conditions since ancient times. The Egyptians prized it highly as a health and diet food because artichokes "cleaned the blood."

Allergies
Alzheimer's Disease
Arthritis/Joint Pain
Atherosclerosis
Blood Pressure
Bursitis
Cancer
Cholesterol
Cramps
Diabetes
Digestion
Fibromyalgia
Gall Stones
Gallbladder

Heart Disease
Hepatitis
Inflammation
Irritable Bowel Syndrome
Kidney Stones
Kidneys
Liver
Obesity
Parkinson's Disease
Pneumonia
Rheumatism
Rosacea
Shingles
Sinus

One medium artichoke has 60 calories, no fat,
7 grams fiber, 13 grams carbohydrates.

Asparagus

The National Cancer Institute states that asparagus is one of the top-notch foods on their lists for helping the body to fight cancer. Along with containing the phyto-chemical glutathione, asparagus is high in rutin which is a recognized aid in strengthening blood vessels.

Aging
Alzheimer's Disease
Anemia
Arthritis/Joint Pain
Atherosclerosis
Blood Pressure
Bronchitis
Cancer
Cervical Cancer
Cholesterol
Colon
Colon Cancer
Constipation
Depression
Diabetes
Diverticulitis
Emphysema
Eyes
Fibromyalgia
Fingernails/Hair
Gall Stones

Heart Disease
Heartburn
Hepatitis
Immune System
Inflammation
Irritable Bowel Syndrome
Kidneys
Liver
Lung Cancer
Lungs
Lupus
Menopause
Multiple Sclerosis
Muscles/Ligaments
Nervousness
Obesity
Parkinson's Disease
Phlegm
Premenstrual Syndrome
Prostate
Rheumatism

Rosacea	Teeth/Gums
Shingles	Thyroid/Goiter
Stress	Urinary Tract
Stroke	Varicose Veins

Four medium asparagus spears have 13 calories, no fat,
1 gram fiber, 2 grams carbohydrates.

Avocados

Hass avocados (the most common variety) contain several different phytonutrients which have been proven to target multiple signal pathways, leading to an increase of free radicals inside cancerous and pre-cancerous cells in humans: this means that only these cells are damaged, while normal human cells are not.

Other studies by UCLA scientists had already proven in the past that Hass avocados could inhibit the growth of prostate cancer cells, due to their high content in lutein, zeaxanthin, alpha-carotene and beta-carotene. Of these, about 70% is represented by lutein.

Aging
Alzheimer's Disease
Arthritis/Joint Pain
Blood Pressure
Breast Cancer
Bursitis
Cancer
Cholesterol
Circulation
Constipation
Cramps
Diabetes
Energy
Eyes
Fibromyalgia
Fingernails/Hair

Gall Stones
Gallbladder
Heart Disease
Heartburn
Hypoglycemia
Inflammation
Insomnia
Irritable Bowel Syndrome
Liver
Lungs
Lupus
Menopause
Multiple Sclerosis
Muscles/Ligaments
Nervousness
Obesity

Pain	Skin
Parkinson's Disease	Stress
Premenstrual Syndrome	Stroke
Prostate Cancer	Thyroid/Goiter
Shingles	Ulcerative Colitis

One medium avocado has 288 calories, 27 grams fat,
12 grams fiber, 15 grams carbohydrates.

Bananas

Trying to give up smoking? Have a banana. Bananas have B6, B12, potassium and magnesium which help the body recover from nicotine withdrawal effects.

Allergies

Anemia

Arthritis/Joint Pain

Atherosclerosis

Blood Pressure

Cancer

Cholesterol

Colds

Colon

Colon Cancer

Constipation

Cramps

Depression

Diabetes

Diarrhea

Digestion

Diverticulitis

Emphysema

Energy

Eyes

Gout

Heart Disease

Heartburn

Hemorrhoids

Influenza

Insomnia

Irritable Bowel Syndrome

Kidneys

Lungs

Lupus

Menopause

Multiple Sclerosis

Nausea

Nervousness

Obesity

Osteoporosis

Pain

Parkinson's Disease

Premenstrual Syndrome

Shingles

Stress

Stroke

Thyroid/Goiter   Ulcers
Ulcerative Colitis

One medium banana has 105 calories, no fat,
3 grams fiber, 27 grams carbohydrates.

Beans

According to the United States Department of Agriculture's list of 20 high-antioxidant sources of common foods, beans are listed four times. The antioxidants in beans have been linked to lowering the risk of colon and lung cancers.

Acne
Aging
Allergies
Atherosclerosis
Blood Pressure
Blood Sugar
Bursitis
Cancer
Cholesterol
Circulation
Colon
Colon Cancer
Constipation
Cramps
Depression
Diabetes
Diverticulitis
Energy
Eyes
Fingernails/Hair
Gallbladder

Headache
Heart Disease
Hemorrhoids
Hepatitis
Hypoglycemia
Immune System
Inflammation
Kidneys
Liver
Lung Cancer
Lungs
Menopause
Multiple Sclerosis
Muscles/Ligaments
Nervousness
Obesity
Osteoporosis
Pain
Pancreas
Parkinson's Disease
Pneumonia

Premenstrual Syndrome

Prostate

Rheumatism

Shingles

Sinus

Stress

Stroke

Thyroid/Goiter

Ulcers

Urinary Tract

Varicose Veins

One cup black beans has 227 calories, 1 gram fat,
15 grams fiber, 41 grams carbohydrates.

Once cup garbanzo beans has 268 calories, 4 grams fat,
12 grams fiber, 45 grams carbohydrates.

Beets

A United Kingdom study, which was published in the American Heart Association journal, 'Hypertension', stated that beetroot juice significantly lowers blood pressure. This study was conducted at the William Harvey Research Institute – the same institute that discovered that aspirin prevents heart attacks and stroke.

Alzheimer's Disease

Anemia

Asthma

Blood Pressure

Bronchitis (especially beet greens)

Cancer

Cholesterol

Circulation

Colon

Colon Cancer

Constipation

Diabetes

Diarrhea (especially beet greens)

Digestion

Diverticulitis

Emphysema

Energy

Eyes

Fibromyalgia

Gallbladder (especially beet greens)

Gas (especially beet greens)

Gout (especially beet greens)

Heart Disease

Hemorrhoids

Hepatitis

Inflammation

Insomnia

Irritable Bowel Syndrome

Liver

Lung Cancer

Menopause

Multiple Sclerosis

Muscles/Ligaments

Nervousness

Obesity

Osteoporosis

Pain

Parkinson's Disease

Phlegm

Pneumonia

Premenstrual Syndrome

Prostate

Rosacea

Shingles (especially
    beet greens)

Sinus

Skin

Skin Cancer

Stroke

Varicose Veins

One cup beets has 58 calories, no fat,
4 grams fiber, 13 grams carbohydrates.

Blackberries

Blackberries have been used medicinally throughout history. Ancient Greeks and Europeans discovered that blackberries effectively treated gout. In the Middle East, the leaves have been used in a tea to treat bleeding gum for over two thousand years. Native Americans used blackberry root tea to cure diarrhea.

Allergies	Lupus
Alzheimer's Disease	Multiple Sclerosis
Asthma	Muscles/Ligaments
Constipation	Nervousness
Diarrhea	Obesity
Energy	Pain
Gall Stones	Parkinson's Disease
Gallbladder	Rosacea
Gout	Shingles
Hemorrhoids	Sinus
Hepatitis	Skin
Hypoglycemia	Stress
Immune System	Stroke
Inflammation	Ulcerative Colitis
Irritable Bowel Syndrome	Ulcers
Kidneys	Varicose Veins
Liver	

One cup blackberries has 61 calories, 1 grams fat,
8 grams fiber, 14 grams carbohydrates.

Blackcurrants

Studies done at the Scottish Crop Research Institute revealed that blackcurrants, rich in an anti-oxidant called anthocyanins, are the healthiest of all the berries. These compounds help ward off health problems like heart disease, cancer, Alzheimer's Disease, diabetes, liver problems and even bladder stones.

Alzheimer's Disease	Hepatitis
Blood Pressure	Inflammation
Cancer	Influenza
Circulation	Insomnia
Colds	Kidneys
Diabetes	Liver
Diarrhea	Multiple Sclerosis
Energy	Muscles/Ligaments
Eyes	Pain
Gallbladder	Thyroid/Goiter
Heart Disease	Ulcers

One cup blackcurrants has 70 calories,
no fat, no fiber, 17 grams carbohydrates.

Blueberries

"When it comes to brain protection, there's nothing quite like blueberries, according to Tufts neuroscientist James Joseph," as recounted in Newsweek (6/17/02). "Call the blueberry the brain berry", says Joseph, who attributes the effects to its antioxidant and anti-inflammatory compounds. In the Wall Street Journal (4/29/03), a recent article on reversing memory loss noted "blueberries . . . had the strongest impact" in a study showing aging rodents behaved more like their younger counterparts when fed several different fruits. Want to have good memory? Eat blueberries!

Aging	Eyes
Allergies	Fibromyalgia
Alzheimer's Disease	Gall Stones
Asthma	Gallbladder
Atherosclerosis	Glaucoma
Blood Pressure	Gout
Bronchitis	Heart Disease
Cancer	Hemorrhoids
Colds	Hepatitis
Constipation	Hypoglycemia
Diabetes	Immune System
Diarrhea	Inflammation
Diverticulitis	Irritable Bowel Syndrome
Emphysema	Kidneys
Energy	Liver

Lungs

Lupus

Menopause

Multiple Sclerosis

Muscles/Ligaments

Nervousness

Obesity

Pain

Pancreas

Parkinson's Disease

Rheumatism

Rosacea

Shingles

Sinus

Skin

Stress

Stroke

Ulcerative Colitis

Ulcers

Urinary Tract

Varicose Veins

One cup blueberries has 82 calories, no fat,
3 grams fiber, 21 grams carbohydrates.

Brazil Nuts

Selenium is a powerful antioxidant that works to neutralize free radicals in your body. Brazil nuts are perhaps the richest source of selenium of all foods. Just eating two Brazil nuts a day could help fight against cancer.

Acne

Arthritis/Joint Pain

Cancer

Diabetes

Energy

Eyes

Fibromyalgia

Fingernails/Hair

Gall Stones

Heart Disease

Hepatitis

Multiple Sclerosis

Muscles/Ligaments

Nervousness

Premenstrual Syndrome

Prostate

Shingles

Skin

Skin Cancer

Stress

Thyroid/Goiter

Urinary Tract

One ounce (7 Brazil nuts) has 83 calories,
19 grams fat (4 grams unsaturated),
2 grams fiber, 3 grams carbohydrates.

Broccoli

In February, 2000, the 'American Journal of Clinical Nutrition' published a paper that listed foods most likely to prevent colon cancer. The food that stood out the most was broccoli.

Acne

Aging

Allergies

Alzheimer's Disease

Anemia

Arthritis/Joint Pain

Asthma

Atherosclerosis

Blood Pressure

Breast Cancer

Bronchitis

Bursitis

Cancer

Cervical Cancer

Circulation

Colds

Colon

Colon Cancer

Constipation

Cramps

Depression

Diabetes

Diverticulitis

Emphysema

Energy

Esophageal Cancer

Eyes

Fibromyalgia

Fingernails/Hair

Gall Stones

Gastrointestinal Cancer

Headache

Heart Disease

Heartburn

Hemorrhoids

Hepatitis

Hypoglycemia

Immune System

Inflammation

Influenza

Kidneys

Liver

Lung Cancer

Lungs

Lupus

Menopause

Multiple Sclerosis

Muscles/Ligaments

Nervousness

Obesity

Osteoporosis

Pain

Pancreas

Pancreatic Cancer

Parkinson's Disease

Pneumonia

Premenstrual Syndrome

Prostate

Rectal Cancer

Rheumatism

Rosacea

Shingles

Sinus

Stomach Cancer

Stress

Stroke

Teeth/Gums

Varicose Veins

One cup broccoli has 29 calories, no fat,
2 grams fiber, 6 grams carbohydrates

"When you're green inside, you're clean inside."

—Dr. Bernard Jensen

Brown Rice

Researchers have found that eating five or more servings of white rice per week was associated with an increased risk of type 2 diabetes. In contrast, eating two or more servings of brown rice per week was associated with a lower risk of type 2 diabetes.

Acne

Aging

Allergies

Anemia

Arthritis/Joint Pain

Atherosclerosis

Bursitis

Cancer

Colds

Colon

Constipation

Depression

Diabetes

Diarrhea

Digestion

Diverticulitis

Emphysema

Energy

Eyes

Fingernails/Hair

Gall Stones

Gout

Headache

Heart Disease

Heartburn

Hemorrhoids

Hepatitis

Hypoglycemia

Immune System

Influenza

Insomnia

Irritable Bowel Syndrome

Kidneys

Liver

Lungs

Lupus

Menopause

Multiple Sclerosis

Nausea

Nervousness

Obesity

Osteoporosis

Pancreas   Shingles

Parkinson's Disease   Stomach Cancer

Premenstrual Syndrome   Stress

Prostate   Stroke

Rheumatism   Thyroid/Goiter

Rosacea

One cup brown rice has 216 calories, 2 grams fat,
4 grams fiber, 45 grams carbohydrates.

Brussels Sprouts

Research published in the 'International Journal of Cancer' shows that Brussels sprouts protect against the acids that may cause a cancerous bladder. Testing revealed that those who had the highest intake of Brussels sprouts and cruciferous vegetables had a 29% lower risk of a cancerous bladder than those who ate the least.

Acne

Aging

Allergies

Alzheimer's Disease

Anemia

Arthritis/Joint Pain

Asthma

Atherosclerosis

Breast Cancer

Bursitis

Cancer

Colds

Colon

Colon Cancer

Constipation

Cramps

Depression

Diverticulitis

Emphysema

Esophageal Cancer

Eyes

Fibromyalgia

Fingernails/Hair

Gall Stones

Hypoglycemia

Inflammation

Kidneys

Liver

Lungs

Lupus

Multiple Sclerosis

Muscles/Ligaments

Obesity

Pancreas

Pancreatic Cancer

Pneumonia

Rheumatism

Rosacea

Shingles   Stress

Sinus   Stroke

One cup Brussels sprouts has 37 calories,
no fat, 3 grams fiber, 8 grams carbohydrates.

"Nutrition can be compared with a chain in which all essential items are separate links. We know what happens if one link of a chain is weak or is missing. The whole chain falls apart."

Patrick Wright, Ph.D.

Buckwheat Germ

Did you know that buckwheat is not a grain? It actually is a fruit seed that is related to sorrel, making it a good substitute for people who are sensitive to wheat.

Aging

Asthma

Blood Pressure

Cancer

Colon

Colon Cancer

Constipation

Diabetes

Digestion

Gout

Heart Disease

Hemorrhoids

Immune System

Influenza

Kidneys

Liver

Lung Cancer

Lungs

Multiple Sclerosis

Nervousness

Obesity

Pain

Shingles

Ulcers

Varicose Veins

One cup buckwheat germ has 583 calories, 6 grams fat,
17 grams fiber, 122 grams carbohydrates.

Cabbage

The ancient Greeks believed in the curative power of cabbage. Hippocrates often prescribed it boiled with salt for patients with violent colic. Pythagoras even composed several entire books on the virtues of cabbage. It was said that Diogenes ate cabbage on the recommendation of Pythagoras while Arisstippus, another Greek philosopher, refused to even have it in his kitchen. Maybe it's just a coincidence but Diogenes lived to the ripe old age of 90 and Arrisstippus died at the age of 40.

Acne	Diarrhea
Aging	Digestion
Allergies	Diverticulitis
Alzheimer's Disease	Esophageal Cancer
Arthritis/Joint Pain	Eyes
Asthma	Gout
Blood Pressure	Heart Disease
Breast Cancer	Heartburn
Bronchitis	Hemorrhoids
Cancer	Hepatitis
Cervical Cancer	Hypoglycemia
Colon	Immune System
Colon Cancer	Inflammation
Constipation	Influenza
Cramps	Insomnia
Depression	Kidneys
Diabetes	Liver

Lung Cancer	Pancreatic Cancer
Lungs	Prostate
Lupus	Rosacea
Menopause	Shingles
Multiple Sclerosis	Sinus
Muscles/Ligaments	Stress
Nervousness	Teeth/Gums
Obesity	Ulcers
Pain	Urinary Tract
Pancreas	Uterine Cancer

One cup cabbage has 16 calories, no fat,
2 grams fiber, 4 grams carbohydrates.

Cantaloupe

Do you need to protect yourself from second hand smoke? Richard Baybutt, associate professor of nutrition at Kansas State, discovered that a common carcinogen in cigarette smoke significantly reduces vitamin A but by adding vitamin A rich food back in your diet, such as cantaloupe, you can counter the negative aspects of smoke - preventing such diseases as emphysema and lung cancer. A diet rich in Vitamin A could explain why some smokers live to be 90.

Acne	Immune System
Alzheimer's Disease	Inflammation
Arthritis/Joint Pain	Irritable Bowel Syndrome
Asthma	Lungs
Blood Pressure	Lupus
Bronchitis	Menopause
Bursitis	Multiple Sclerosis
Cancer	Muscles/Ligaments
Cholesterol	Obesity
Cramps	Pain
Diverticulitis	Pancreas
Eyes	Parkinson's Disease
Gall Stones	Pneumonia
Gallbladder	Rosacea
Gout	Skin
Heart Disease	Stress
Hemorrhoids	Teeth/Gums
Hepatitis	Ulcerative Colitis

One medium cantaloupe has 187 calories, 1 gram fat,
5 grams fiber, 45 grams carbohydrates.

Carrots

The carrot, rich in carotenoids, was the star of six epidemiological studies that looked at the association of carotenoids and cancer. The findings reported that cartenoids not only reduced cancer, but heart disease as well. In one study of 1300 elderly persons in Massachusetts, those who had at least one serving of carrots (and/ or squash) each day had a 60% reduction in their risk of heart attacks compared to those who ate less than one serving a day.

Acne	Diarrhea
Aging	Digestion
Allergies	Diverticulitis
Alzheimer's Disease	Emphysema
Anemia	Esophageal Cancer
Asthma	Eyes
Atherosclerosis	Fibromyalgia
Blood Presssure	Fingernails/Hair
Breast Cancer	Gall Stones
Bronchitis	Gallbladder
Bursitis	Gas
Cancer	Gout
Cervical Cancer	Headache
Circulation	Heart Disease
Colds	Heartburn
Colon	Hemorrhoids
Colon Cancer	Hepatitis
Constipation	Hypoglycemia
Diabetes	Immune System

Inflammation

Influenza

Insomnia

Irritable Bowel Syndrome

Kidneys

Liver

Lung Cancer

Lungs

Menopause

Multiple Sclerosis

Muscles/Ligaments

Obesity

Osteoporosis

Pain

Pancreas

Parkinson's Disease

Phlegm

Pneumonia

Premenstrual Syndrome

Prostate

Prostate Cancer

Rheumatism

Rosacea

Shingles

Sinus

Skin

Stroke

Teeth/Gums

Thyroid/Goiter

Uterine Cancer

Varicose Veins

One large carrot has 29 calories, no fat,
2 grams fiber, 7 grams carbohydrates.

"An old-fashioned vegetable soup, without any enhancement, is a more powerful anti carcinogen than any known medicine."

—James Duke M.D. (U.S.D.A.)

Cauliflower

Although cauliflower looks like a vegetable, it's really the flower of the plant. In fact, in the early days of England, it was referred to as flowered cabbage – hence the name. This high vitamin C "flower" has been linked to the prevention of many cancers – including breast cancer and lung cancer.

Aging	Hypoglycemia
Allergies	Immune System
Arthritis/Joint Pain	Inflammation
Asthma	Kidneys
Blood Pressure (high)	Liver
Breast Cancer	Lung Cancer
Bruises	Lungs
Cancer	Menopause
Colds	Multiple Sclerosis
Colon	Muscles/Ligaments
Colon Cancer	Obesity
Constipation	Osteoporosis
Cramps	Pain
Depression	Pancreas
Diabetes	Pancreatic Cancer
Energy	Parkinson's Disease
Esophageal Cancer	Phlegm
Heart Disease	Prostate
Hepatitis	Prostate Cancer

Rosacea   Teeth/Gums

Stroke

One cup cauliflower has 25 calories, no fat,
3 grams fiber, 5 grams carbohydrates.

Celery

Celery has been used medicinally as a calming agent since early times. Studies have shown that it helps insomnia. The ancient Chinese physicians realized that celery also lowers blood pressure. Ancient Egyptians prescribed celery for rheumatism. Hippocrates also knew the calming power of celery since he often prescribed it to fight inflammation.

Anemia

Arthritis/Joint Pain

Asthma

Blood Pressure

Bronchitis

Bursitis

Cancer

Colds

Colon

Colon Cancer

Constipation

Diverticulitis

Emphysema

Energy

Eyes

Fibromyalgia

Gall Stones

Gallbladder

Gout

Headache

Hepatitis

Hypoglycemia

Inflammation

Influenza

Insomnia

Irritable Bowel Syndrome

Kidneys

Muscles/Ligaments

Nervousness

Obesity

Pain

Pancreas

Phlegm

Pneumonia

Premenstrual Syndrome

Rheumatism

Rosacea

Shingles

Sinus   Ulcers

Stomach Cancer   Urinary Tract

Teeth/Gums

One celery stalk has 8 calories, no fat
1 gram fiber, 2 grams carbohydrates

Cherries

In 2008, the University of Michigan conducted a study on the health benefits of cherries. Due to the powerful antioxidants in cherries, known as anthocyanins, they concluded that a diet rich in cherries may help lower body fat, total weight, inflammation and cholesterol – all major risks for heart disease.

Acne

Aging

Alzheimer's Disease

Arthritis/Joint Pain

Atherosclerosis

Cancer

Cholesterol

Colds

Diabetes

Diverticulitis

Emphysema

Eyes

Gall Stones

Gas

Gout

Headache

Heart Disease

Hemorrhoids

Hypoglycemia

Inflammation

Insomnia

Irritable Bowel Syndrome

Kidneys

Liver

Multiple Sclerosis

Obesity

Pain

Pancreas

Rheumatism

Stroke

Thyroid/Goiter

Urinary Tract

Varicose Veins

One cherry has 3 calories, no fat,
no fiber, 1 gram carbohydrates.

*"The art of medicine consists in amusing
the patient while nature cures the disease."*

—Voltaire

Coconut

Can something as simple as coconut oil build your immune system? According to a study done by Dr. Conrado Dayrit it certainly can be effective. He tested 14 HIV infected individuals by giving them a dose of 3 tablespoons of coconut oil daily. With no other antiviral used, within six months, sixty percent of the participants showed noticeable improvement with increased CD4 count, lowered viral load and better overall health.

Acne	Heart Disease
Aging	Hemorrhoids
Asthma	Hepatitis
Bladder	Immune System
Breast Cancer	Influenza
Bronchitis	Kidney Stones
Cancer	Kidneys
Chronic Fatigue Syndrome	Liver
Colds	Nausea
Colon	Obesity
Colon Cancer	Osteoporosis
Constipation	Pancreas
Diabetes	Pneumonia
Digestion	Premenstrual Syndrome
Energy	Skin
Fingernails/Hair	Stress
Gallbladder	Teeth/Gums

Thyroid/Goiter   Urinary Tract
Ulcers

One cup shredded coconut has 283 calories, 27 grams fat,
7 grams fiber, 12 grams carbohydrates.

Collards

Interested in having strong bones? Collard greens may do the trick. Just one cup of collard greens packs a whopping 880% of the daily recommended amount of vitamin K — the vitamin that helps you build strong bones and fight osteoporosis.

Aging

Alzheimer's Disease

Arthritis/Joint Pain

Asthma

Bursitis

Cancer

Circulation

Colds

Constipation

Cramps

Depression

Diabetes

Digestion

Emphysema

Energy

Eyes

Fibromyalgia

Fingernails/Hair

Gas

Headache

Heart Disease

Immune System

Inflammation

Influenza

Insomnia

Irritable Bowel Syndrome

Liver

Lung Cancer

Lungs

Menopause

Multiple Sclerosis

Muscles/Ligaments

Nervousness

Obesity

Osteoporosis

Pancreas

Parkinson's Disease

Pneumonia

Premenstrual Syndrome

Rheumatism

Rosacea   Stroke

Stress   Varicose Veins

One cup collard greens has 10 calories, no fat,
1 gram fiber, 2 grams carbohydrates.

Corn

Corn, a staple in Mexico for over 9000 years, has recently had some interesting studies concerning eye health. Corn contains a high amount of lutein and zeaxanthin. In 1994 Harvard Medical School and Research Center determined that high levels of lutein and zeaxanthin could reduce the risk of age related macular disease by 43%. Further studies at Cornell University showed that heating the corn at 115° Celsius increased the anti-free radical activity by 53%.

Breast Cancer	Insomnia
Cancer	Kidneys
Cholesterol	Lungs
Colds	Pneumonia
Constipation	Premenstrual Syndrome
Energy	Skin
Eyes	Stress

One cup corn has 132 calories, 2 grams fat,
4 grams fiber, 29 grams carbohydrates.

Cranberries

Can cranberries really fight the flu? They can and here's why. Cranberries are a good source of proanthocyanidins, astringent substances that binds to the viruses so they can't attach to cells and cause infection. When the bacteria can't adhere to the cells they are simply flushed out of the body.

Allergies	Nausea
Alzheimer's Disease	Obesity
Blood Pressure	Parkinson's Disease
Colds	Pneumonia
Eyes	Premenstrual Syndrome
Headache	Rosacea
Influenza	Shingles
Kidneys	Ulcers
Liver	Urinary Tract
Lungs	Uterine Cancer
Menopause	

One cup cranberries has 43 calories, no fat,
4 grams fiber, 12 grams carbohydrates.

Cucumbers

Cucumbers, because of their high water content, are natural diuretics. This cleansing action helps to remove the chemical toxins and uric acid that builds up in the body – not only fighting gout but benefiting the kidneys and the joints as well.

Arthritis/Joint Pain
Blood Pressure
Constipation
Digestion
Eyes
Gallbladder
Gout
Hypoglycemia
Inflammation
Insomnia

Kidneys
Menopause
Muscles/Ligaments
Obesity
Pain
Premenstrual Syndrome
Rosacea
Shingles
Teeth/Gums

One cup cucumbers has 14 calories, no fat,
1 gram fiber, 3 grams carbohydrates.

Dates

Dates have been cultivated from ancient times, probably as early as 6000 BC. Because of their rich taste, high sugar content (that provides energy) and the fact that they could be carried in a caravan without spoilage for as long as 18 months, they were considered quite valuable. Caravans heading to Petra and beyond to the Mediterranean coast, traded dates for Frankincense.

Alzheimer's Disease	Lungs
Anemia	Multiple Sclerosis
Cancer	Muscles/Ligaments
Cramps	Nausea
Diarrhea	Obesity
Energy	Pain
Heart Disease	Shingles
Insomnia	Stomach Cancer
Irritable Bowel Syndrome	Thyroid/Goiter

One date has 66 calories, no fat,
2 grams fiber, 18 grams carbohydrates.

"Health requires healthy food."

—Roger Williams, PhD

Eggplant

Thomas Jefferson, an avid experimental botanist, first introduced the eggplant to America in 1806. This purple vegetable is not only gorgeous but is certainly healthy as well. The American Diabetes Association, the National Diabetes Education Program of NIH, and the Mayo Clinic all endorse eggplant in the management of type 2 diabetes because of its high fiber and low soluble content.

Arthritis/Joint Pain

Blood Pressure

Cancer

Cholesterol

Circulation

Colds

Diabetes

Diverticulitis

Kidneys

Nervousness

Pneumonia

Stroke

One cup eggplant has 19 calories, no fat,
3 grams fiber, 5 grams carbohydrates.

Eggs

Are eggs good or bad for you? Good, says Harvard Medical School. In the 'Harvard Heart Letter', July 2006, they stated that not only are they good for you (in moderation) but they are a good source of nutrients...especially choline which has been linked with preserving memory, and lutein and zeaxanthin which may protect against vision loss.

Alzheimer's Disease	Multiple Sclerosis
Anemia	Muscles/Ligaments
Colds	Nausea
Depression	Nervousness
Energy	Obesity
Eyes	Osteoporosis
Fingernails/Hair	Parkinson's Disease
Gout	Pneumonia
Heartburn	Prostate
Immune System	Rheumatism
Insomnia	Shingles
Lungs	Stress
Lupus	Thyroid/Goiter
Menopause	

One large egg has 73 calories, 5 grams fat,
no fiber, no carbohydrates

Figs

Figs were promoted for health back in 60 BC when Plato recommended that athletes eat them daily to boost their energy and to prevent leg cramps. It's no surprise then that the Greeks restricted their export so their athletes would have the advantage at the Olympic Games.

Anemia	Hemorrhoids
Blood Pressure	Irritable Bowel Syndrome
Colon	Lungs
Colon Cancer	Multiple Sclerosis
Constipation	Muscles/Ligaments
Cramps	Obesity
Energy	Pain
Gallbladder	Stroke

One medium fig has 37 calories, no fat,
1 gram fiber, 10 grams carbohydrates.

"Unless we put medical freedom into the Constitution, the time will come when medicine will organize into an undercover dictatorship to restrict the art of healing to one class of men and deny equal privileges to others; the Constitution of the Republic should make a special privilege for medical freedoms as well as religious freedom."

—Benjamin Rush, MD.
A signer of the Declaration of Independence
and personal physician to George Washington

Fish: (Salmon, Tuna, Sardines)

All fat is bad for you, right? Wrong. There's bad fat such as Omega 6 - that clogs up your arteries and then there's good fat – Omega 3 fatty acids - that actually help prevent heart disease. In the 1970's a study of Inuit indians in Greenland, who had a diet rich in fish and marine life, revealed that the Inuits had very little heart disease or diabetes. The study determined that it was due to Omega – 3. They also discovered that their ratio of good fat Omega -3) to bad fat (Omega – 6) was 1:1, which is ideal. With American's junk food diet, the ratio is as high as 50:1. The way to counter act that is to add Omega-3 regularly into your diet. Fish such as salmon, tuna and sardines are loaded with omega 3 fatty acids.

Acne	Colds
Aging	Colon
Allergies	Colon Cancer
Alzheimer's Disease	Cramps
Anemia	Depression
Arthritis/Joint Pain/Joint Pain	Diabetes
Asthma	Diverticulitis
Atherosclerosis	Energy
Blood Pressure	Eyes
Bronchitis	Fibromyalgia
Bursitis	Fingernails/Hair
Cancer	Gallbladder
Cholesterol	Gas
Circulation	Gout

Headache

Heart Disease

Heartburn

Hemorrhoids

Hepatitis

Hypoglycemia

Immune System

Inflammation

Influenza

Insomnia

Irritable Bowel Syndrome

Liver

Lungs

Lupus

Menopause

Multiple Sclerosis

Muscles/Ligaments

Nervousness

Obesity

Osteoporosis

Pain

Parkinson's Disease

Pneumonia

Premenstrual Syndrome

Prostate

Rheumatism

Shingles

Sinus

Skin

Skin Cancer

Stress

Stroke

Sinus

Teeth/Gums

Thyroid/Goiter

Ulcerative Colitis

Urinary Tract

Three ounces salmon has 142 calories,
7 grams fat (1 gram saturated),
no fiber, no carbohydrates.

Three ounces tuna has 91 calories, 1 gram fat,
no fiber, no carbohydrates.

Two sardines canned in oil) have 49 calories,
3 grams fat, no fiber, no carbohydrates.

Flax/Flaxseeds

In 1992, a study on the health benefits specific to heart disease was conducted by Holly A. Dieken of the Food and Nutrition Department at North Dakota State University. Two groups of people – one group with normal cholesterol and one group with high cholesterol were give two flaxseed muffins a day (containing a total of 5 ½ tablespoons of flaxseeds.) The normal subjects showed no change in their cholesterol levels, but those with high cholesterol dropped their blood serum triglycerides by 17 percent revealing a definite heart healthy benefit.

Acne	Constipation
Aging	Cramps
Allergies	Depression
Alzheimer's Disease	Diabetes
Arthritis/Joint Pain	Digestion
Asthma	Emphysema
Atherosclerosis	Energy
Blood Pressure	Eyes
Breast Cancer	Fingernails/Hair
Bronchitis	Gall Stones
Bursitis	Gallbladder
Cancer	Gas
Cholesterol	Gout
Circulation	Heart Disease
Colon	Hemorrhoids
Colon Cancer	Hepatitis

Immune System

Inflammation

Irritable Bowel Syndrome

Kidney Stones

Kidneys

Liver

Lungs

Lupus

Menopause

Mental Health

Multiple Sclerosis

Muscles/Ligaments

Nervousness

Obesity

Osteoporosis

Pain

Pancreatic Cancer

Parkinson's Disease

Premenstrual Syndrome

Prostate

Prostate Cancer

Rheumatism

Rosacea

Shingles

Skin

Stroke

Thyroid/Goiter

One tablespoon flax seeds has 59 calories, 4 grams fat,
3 grams fiber, 4 grams carbohydrates.

Grapefruit

A study done in Israel and published in the 'Journal of Agricultural and Food Chemistry' revealed that antioxidants in grapefruit - especially red grapefruit - may help to lower cholesterol. In a controlled study group of patients with heart disease, the scientists gave only some of the participants ½ grapefruit a day. At the end of the study those who ate the grapefruit showed significantly reduced levels of cholesterol.

Acne
Allergies
Alzheimer's Disease
Arthritis/Joint Pain
Asthma
Atherosclerosis
Blood Pressure
Bursitis
Cancer
Cholesterol
Circulation
Colds
Colon
Colon Cancer
Cramps
Diabetes
Diverticulitis
Emphysema

Eyes
Gall Stones
Heart Disease
Immune System
Inflammation
Influenza
Kidneys
Liver
Menopause
Multiple Sclerosis
Obesity
Osteoporosis
Pain
Pancreas
Parkinson's Disease
Phlegm
Pneumonia
Premenstrual Syndrome

Prostate	Sinus
Prostate Cancer	Stomach Cancer
Rheumatism	Stress
Rosacea	Stroke
Shingles	Varicose Veins

One cup grapefruit has 85 calories, no fat,
no fiber, 22 grams carbohydrates.

"This illustrates the need for modern medicine and science to turn its attention to the plant world once again to find new medicine that might cure cancer, AIDS, diabetes, and many other diseases and conditions."

—Norman R. Farnsworth, Ph.D.,
Professor of Pharmacology
at the University of Illinois at Chicago

Grapes

According to the Linus Pauling Institute at Oregon State University, the compound resveratrol has been found to exert a number of potentially cardioprotective effects. So how much resveratrol is found in grapes or in a glass of wine? They state that one cup of red table grapes provides between .24 and 1.25 mg of resveratrol - similar to one 5 ounce glass of red wine, which provides between 30 and 1.07 mg. Wine, grape juice or table grapes, this fruit is definitely heart healthy.

Aging	Fibromyalgia
Allergies	Gall Stones
Alzheimer's Disease	Gallbladder
Anemia	Gas
Atherosclerosis	Gout
Blood Pressure	Heart Disease
Bronchitis	Heartburn
Cancer	Hepatitis
Circulation	Inflammation
Colds	Kidneys
Colon	Lung Cancer
Colon Cancer	Lungs
Constipation	Menopause
Diverticulitis	Muscles/Ligaments
Emphysema	Nausea (grape juice)
Energy	Obesity
Eyes	Osteoporosis

Pain   Shingles
Pancreas   Skin
Prostate   Stomach Cancer
Rheumatism   Thyroid/Goiter
Rosacea   Varicose Veins

One cup grapes has 61 calories, no fat,
1 gram fiber, 16 grams carbohydrates.

Green Tea

Why is green tea so good for you? It's rich in polyphenols, the antioxidant that helps build your immune system. Many studies have been done both in the laboratory and with group test studies and the results have been remarkable. The University of Maryland Medical School quotes one study of 472 women with various stages of breast cancer who were asked to drink green tea daily. Researchers found that women who consumed the most green tea experienced the least spread of cancer - and even more amazing, those who drank at least five cups a day were less likely to suffer recurrences of the disease after completion of treatment.

Allergies

Arthritis/Joint Pain

Asthma

Breast Cancer

Cancer

Cholesterol

Circulation

Colds

Colon

Colon Cancer

Diarrhea

Diverticulitis

Emphysema

Esophageal Cancer

Gout

Heart Disease

Immune System

Inflammation

Influenza

Kidneys

Liver

Lungs

Multiple Sclerosis

Muscles/Ligaments

Nausea

Nervousness

Obesity

Pancreas

Pancreatic Cancer

Parkinson's Disease

Pneumonia

Prostate

Prostate Cancer

Sinus

Skin

Skin Cancer

Stomach Cancer

Stroke

Teeth/Gums

Ulcers

Urinary Tract

Varicose Veins

One cup green tea has 2 calories, no fat
no fiber, no carbohydrates.

Honey

Hippocrates said, "Honey serves food, health and energy" and suggested the Greek athletes use it before games to give them the strength and energy they needed. Many studies have been done to verify this fact. At the University of Memphis researchers did a study on the benefits of honey in sporting events. Their conclusion was that, unlike sugar which gives you quick energy and then falls off, the honey gave the participants sustained energy for two hours. Why? Due to the fact that honey has tremendous vitamins and minerals and sugar has virtually none. Especially important is that sugar has 2 mg. of potassium, where the honey packs a powerhouse of 52 mg.

Allergies	Insomnia
Anemia	Liver
Asthma	Lungs
Blood Pressure	Nausea
Bronchitis	Obesity
Colds	Osteoporosis
Colon	Phlegm
Digestion	Pneumonia
Energy	Rheumatism
Heart Disease	Sinus
Heartburn	Ulcers
Influenza	

One tablespoon honey has 63 calories, no fat,
no fiber, 17 grams carbohydrates.

"For every drug that benefits a patient, there is a natural substance that can achieve the same effect." —

"Pfeiffer's Law"
—Dr. Carl C. Pfeiffer, M.D., PhD.

Kale

Kale was so plentiful throughout the British Isles that young people made of game of "pullin' the kale" to see what kind of a mate they would have – the amount of dirt clinging to the root was the amount of wealth they would have; the shape, straight or curved, was the shape of their mate's spine and if the taste was bitter, it meant a bitter mate. Robert Burns in his poem, "Halloween," describes young people running into the fields, blindfolded, to select their plants on "that night, when fairies light." Kale may not have fortune telling power, but it certainly has health power. It has seven times the beta carotene as broccoli and ten times the lutein . Additionally kale has the phytochemical, sulforaphane. The 'Journal of Nutrition' in 2004 stated that sulforaphane helps stops breast cancer proliferation. All hail Kale!

Acne	Colon Cancer
Aging	Constipation
Allergies	Cramps
Alzheimer's Disease	Depression
Anemia	Diabetes
Asthma	Diverticulitis
Atherosclerosis	Emphysema
Breast Cancer	Energy
Bronchitis	Esophageal Cancer
Cancer	Eyes
Colds	Fibromyalgia
Colon	Fingernails/Hair

Gall Stones

Gas

Gout

Headache

Heart Disease

Hemorrhoids

Hepatitis

Hypoglycemia

Immune System

Inflammation

Influenza

Insomnia

Irritable Bowel Syndrome

Kidneys

Liver

Lungs

Lupus

Menopause

Multiple Sclerosis

Muscles/Ligaments

Nervousness

Obesity

Osteoporosis

Pain

Pancreas

Parkinson's Disease

Prostate

Rheumatism

Rosacea

Shingles

Sinus

Skin

Stress

Stroke

Ulcers

Varicose Veins

One cup kale has 33 calories, no fat,
1 gram fiber, 7 grams carbohydrates.

Kiwi

Do you suffer from asthma? Kiwi may help the illness. The April, 2004 issue of 'Thorax' cited a study of 18,737 children living in Central and Northern Italy, who were given citrus and kiwifruit (5-7 servings per week). Some had asthma, some did not. The result of the study showed those with asthma benefitted the most with shortness of breath reduced by 37%; severe wheeze reduced by 41%, night time cough reduced by 25% and runny noses reduced by 28%. Vitamin C may be the answer since one kiwi provides117% of the recommended daily allowance.

Acne

Arthritis/Joint Pain

Asthma

Atherosclerosis

Blood Pressure

Bursitis

Circulation

Colds

Constipation

Cramps

Depression

Emphysema

Eyes

Fibromyalgia

Gall Stones

Gas

Immune System

Inflammation

Irritable Bowel Syndrome

Multiple Sclerosis

Obesity

Pain

Pancreas

Parkinson's Disease

Rheumatism

Rosacea

Shingles

Stress

Stroke

Teeth/Gums

One medium kiwi has 46 calories, no fat, 2 grams fiber,
11 grams carbohydrates (+117% MDR of vitamin C)

Lemons/Limes

Do lemons and limes really help fight cancer? In laboratory studies and tests with human cells the compound found in lemons and limes called limonoids have been shown to fight cancers of the mouth, skin, lungs, breast, stomach and colon. Recently the US Agricultural Research Service determined that our bodies can readily absorb these liminoids in lemons and limes and once absorbed this cancer-fighting agent, limonin, can stay in the body for a very long time.

Acne

Aging

Allergies

Alzheimer's Disease

Anemia

Arthritis/Joint Pain

Atherosclerosis

Blood Pressure

Breast Cancer

Cancer

Cholesterol

Circulation

Colds

Colon Cancer

Constipation

Depression

Diabetes

Emphysema

Eyes

Fibromyalgia

Gall Stones

Gallbladder

Gout

Heart Disease

Hepatitis

Inflammation

Influenza

Insomnia

Liver

Lung Cancer

Menopause

Multiple Sclerosis

Muscles/Ligaments

Nausea

Obesity   Sinus

Phlegm   Skin

Pneumonia   Skin Cancer

Premenstrual Syndrome   Stress

Prostate   Stroke

Rheumatism   Stomach Cancer

Shingles   Varicose Veins

One medium lemon has 16 calories, no fat,
2 grams fiber, 5 grams carbohydrates.

One medium lime has 20 calories, no fat,
2 grams fiber, 7 grams carbohydrates.

Lentils

Study after study proves the connection between nutrition and heart disease. In a worldwide study 16,000 men were tested for cardiovascular risk by diet. It was concluded that people, from southern Europe, who ate the most vegetables, especially legumes – like lentils – and fish had a whopping 82% reduction in risk. In yet another study published in the 'Archives of Internal Medicine', a group of 10,000 Americans were tested on their diets for 19 years and once again the finding was that eating high fiber foods, like lentils, helps prevent heart disease.

Acne	Gall Stones
Aging	Heart Disease
Anemia	Inflammation
Arthritis/Joint Pain	Insomnia
Atherosclerosis	Irritable Bowel Syndrome
Blood Pressure	Lung Cancer
Cancer	Multiple Sclerosis
Cholesterol	Muscles/Ligaments
Circulation	Nervousness
Colon	Obesity
Colon Cancer	Parkinson's Disease
Constipation	Premenstrual Syndrome
Diabetes	Rheumatism
Diverticulitis	Rosacea
Fibromyalgia	Stress
Fingernails/Hair	Thyroid/Goiter

Urinary Tract   Varicose Veins

One cup lentils have 229 calories, 1 gram fat,
16 grams fiber, 40 grams carbohydrates.

Mango

According to a study by Texas AgriLife Research lab, food scientists found that mango has been found to prevent or stop cancer – specifically colon and breast cancer cells. Dr. Susanne Talcott, who with her husband, Dr. Steve Talcott, stated that, "It has about four to five times less antioxidant capacity than an average wine grape, and it still holds up fairly well in anticancer activity. If you look at it from the physiological and nutritional standpoint, taking everything together, it would be a high-ranking super food," she said. "It would be good to include mango as part of the regular diet."

Alzheimer's Disease	Kidneys
Arthritis/Joint Pain	Liver
Atherosclerosis	Lungs
Blood Pressure	Multiple Sclerosis
Breast Cancer	Muscles/Ligaments
Cancer	Obesity
Colds	Pain
Colon	Rosacea
Colon Cancer	Shingles
Constipation	Sinus
Digestion	Skin
Emphysema	Thyroid/Goiter
Eyes	

One cup mangoes has 107 calories, no fat,
3 grams fiber, 28 grams carbohydrates.

Mushrooms

Mushrooms can actually bolster your immune system. The Kansai Medical University in Osaka, Japan discovered that the mushroom compound, AHCC, increases the immune system by increasing the dentric cells (DCs) which carry out a key role in a healthy immune system. Their study indicated that the use of AHCC could reduce our need for antibiotics and lessen our rate of bacterial resistance, allowing us to fight infection more easily. AHCC is currently used in Japan as a supplement to ward off infection and maintain a healthy lifestyle.

Arthritis/Joint Pain
Blood Pressure
Bronchitis
Cancer
Cholesterol
Colds
Diverticulitis
Hypoglycemia
Immune System
Inflammation
Influenza
Insomnia
Irritable Bowel Syndrome

Kidneys
Lungs
Multiple Sclerosis
Muscles/Ligaments
Nervousness
Obesity
Osteoporosis
Pain
Pancreas
Prostate
Teeth/Gums
Thyroid/Goiter

One cup mushrooms has 21 calories, no fat,
1 gram fiber, 3 grams carbohydrates.

"We need a paradigm shift, and I think it's beginning to occur. Nutrition needs to be looked at, not as a means of preventing specific deficiency diseases, but as a means of contributing to the overall health of the person and his or her resistance to chronic diseases… This is going to produce a big upsurge in human health in the next twenty years."

—Richard P. Huemer, M.D

Oats

Can oats help memory? Possibly. Throughout the years, there have been numerous studies on the benefits of oats especially in the fight against heart disease, but a new study is currently being undertaken on oats and how it can help Alzheimer's disease. The University of South Australia's Nutritional Physiology Research Centre is investigating whether an oat extract can improve cognitive performance in older adults. "In recent years, there has been growing interest in the use of foods to enhance cognition, (and) with the proportion of Australia's ageing population set to increase over the next several decades, mental disability through age-related cognitive decline looms as a major public health problem with enormous economic and social impact," said research Professor Peter Howe.

Acne	Digestion
Aging	Diverticulitis
Alzheimer's Disease	Energy
Atherosclerosis	Esophageal Cancer
Blood Pressure	Eyes
Bursitis	Gall Stones
Cancer	Headache
Cholesterol	Heart Disease
Colds	Hemorrhoids
Colon / Colon Cancer	Heartburn
Constipation	Hepatitis
Depression	Hypoglycemia
Diabetes	Immune System

Inflammation

Influenza

Insomnia

Lungs

Lupus

Multiple Sclerosis

Muscles/Ligaments

Nausea

Nervousness

Obesity

Osteoporosis

Pancreas

Parkinson's Disease

Premenstrual Syndrome

Rosacea

Shingles

Skin

Stomach Cancer

Stroke

Thyroid/Goiter

Ulcers

Urinary Tract

Varicose Veins

One cup oats has 606 calories, 11 grams fat (2 grams saturated), 17 grams fiber, 103 grams carbohydrates

Okra

Okra, affectionately known as 'that slimy vegetable', is really a powerhouse of nutrients and is helpful in the treatment of diabetic nephropathy, a kidney disease that can follow diabetes. Liu Ke-hu of China's The First Hospital of Jilin University reports that eating okra can reduce the risk of diabetic nephropathy. According to a study published in the October 2005 issue of 'Jilin Medical Journal', Liu and her colleagues split a group of 70 diabetics into two groups. One group received traditional diabetic treatment while the other received the same treatment while eating okra every day. The group that ate okra had better kidney health over six months compared to the control group.

Anemia	Kidneys
Cancer	Liver
Colon	Obesity
Colon Cancer	Osteoporosis
Gallbladder	Parkinson's Disease
Gas	Phlegm
Heart Disease	Rosacea
Irritable Bowel Syndrome	Shingles

One cup okra has 31 calories, no fat,
3 grams fiber, 7 grams carbohydrates.

Olive Oil

The Mediterranean diet has been studied extensively over the past several years, due to the resident's health and longevity. Many conclusions have been drawn, but the one commonality that this diet shares is the abundance of olive oil. In 2005, the 'European Journal Clinical Investigation' published material from the International Conference on the Healthy Effects of Virgin Olive Oil. Among their findings was that olive oil was protective against heart disease, Alzheimer's disease, blood pressure, diabetes, and cancer and certainly contributes to a long healthy life.

Aging	Inflammation
Alzheimer's Disease	Irritable Bowel Syndrome
Arthritis/Joint	Kidneys
Blood Pressure	Liver
Breast Cancer	Lupus
Bronchitis	Menopause
Cancer	Multiple Sclerosis
Cholesterol	Muscles/Ligaments
Depression	Obesity
Diabetes	Osteoporosis
Emphysema	Pancreas
Eyes	Skin
Gall Stones	Stroke
Gallbladder	Ulcers
Heart Disease	Urinary Tract
Hemorrhoids	

One tablespoon olive oil has 144 calories,
13 grams fat, no fiber, no carbohydrates.

Onions

Quercetin is the antioxidant that helps eliminate free radicals from the body. Onions have twice the quercetin as tea and over three times as much as apples. This powerful antioxidant has been helpful in the fight against cataracts, heart disease, cancer and osteoporosis. A recent study at the University of Bern in Switzerland showed that lab animals who were fed just 1 gram of dry onions a day increased their bone density by 17% and mineral density by 13% compared to animals fed a controlled diet.

Acne	Colon Cancer
Aging	Diverticulitis
Allergies	Emphysema
Alzheimer's Disease	Eyes
Arthritis/Joint Pain	Fibromyalgia
Asthma	Fingernails/Hair
Atherosclerosis	Gout
Blood Pressure	Heart Disease
Breast Cancer	Hemorrhoids
Bronchitis	Hypoglycemia
Bursitis	Immune System
Cancer	Inflammation
Cervical Cancer	Influenza
Cholesterol	Kidneys
Circulation	Liver
Colds	Lungs
Colon	Menopause

Multiple Sclerosis

Muscles/Ligaments

Obesity

Osteoporosis

Pancreas

Phlegm

Premenstrual Syndrome

Prostate

Prostate Cancer

Shingles

Stomach Cancer

Teeth/Gums

Thyroid/Goiter

Uterine Cancer

Varicose Veins

One cup onions has 67 calories, no fat,
2 grams fiber, 16 grams carbohydrates.

Oranges

Want to reduce the risk of kidney stones? Just two cups of orange juice a day may be all the prevention you need. A study published in the British Journal of Nutrition stated that women who drank ½ to 1 liter (approximately 2 cups) of orange juice a day increased both their urinary ph value and their citric acid excretion – both of which significantly reduce the forming of calcium oxalate stones.

Acne

Allergies

Alzheimer's Disease

Anemia

Arthritis/Joint Pain

Asthma

Atherosclerosis

Blood Pressure

Bronchitis

Bursitis

Cancer

Circulation

Colds

Colon

Colon Cancer

Constipation

Cramps

Depression

Diarrhea

Diverticulitis

Emphysema

Eyes

Fingernails/Hair

Gall Stones

Gout

Heart Disease

Hemorrhoids

Hepatitis

Hypoglycemia

Immune System

Inflammation

Influenza (especially orange juice)

Kidney Stones

Liver

Lung Cancer

Lungs

Lupus

Menopause

Multiple Sclerosis

Nausea

Nervousness

Obesity

Osteoporosis

Pain

Pancreas

Phlegm

Pneumonia

Premenstrual Syndrome

Prostate

Rheumatism

Shingles

Sinus

Stomach Cancer

Stress

Stroke

Teeth/Gums

Thyroid/Goiter

Ulcerative Colitis

Uterine Cancer

Varicose Veins

One medium orange has 68 calories, no fat,
3 grams fiber, 18 grams carbohydrates.

Papaya

In many studies papaya continues to prove itself to be effective against many types of cancer. An interesting study took place in Mexico where 14 plant foods were evaluated in their ability to halt breast cancer cell growth. Among these foods were avocado, black spote, fuava, mango, prickly Pears cactus, pineapple, grapes, tomato and papaya. The determination was that only the papaya had a significant effect on stopping breast cancer cell growth.

Alzheimer's Disease
Arthritis/Joint Pain
Asthma
Atherosclerosis
Breast Cancer
Bronchitis
Bursitis
Cancer
Cervical Cancer
Colds
Colon
Colon Cancer
Digestion
Emphysema
Energy
Eyes
Fingernails/Hair

Gallbladder
Gas
Heart Disease
Heartburn
Hemorrhoids
Hepatitis
Immune System
Inflammation
Irritable Bowel Syndrome
Liver
Lung Cancer
Lungs
Multiple Sclerosis
Obesity
Pain
Parkinson's Disease
Prostate

Prostate Cancer   Stress

Rosacea   Ulcerative Colitis

Sinus   Uterine Cancer

Skin

One medium papaya has 118 calories, no fat,
5 grams fiber, 30 grams carbohydrates (+313% MDR of vitamin C).

Peaches

At the Texas AgriLife Research Center, scientists have discovered that peach and plum extracts actually killed breast cancer cells. The tests were done side by side on cancerous cells and normal cells. Not only did the cancerous cells die, but the normal cells were not harmed even with the larger doses of the extracts. Peaches - yet another weapon in the fight against breast cancer.

Allergies
Arthritis/Joint Pain
Atherosclerosis
Breast Cancer
Cancer
Colon
Constipation
Digestion
Diverticulitis
Emphysema
Hemorrhoids
Kidneys
Liver

Lungs
Multiple Sclerosis
Nausea (canned peaches are best)
Nervousness
Obesity
Pain
Pneumonia
Rheumatism
Shingles
Sinus
Skin
Stroke
Ulcerative Colitis

One medium peach has 38 calories, no fat,
1 gram fiber, 9 grams carbohydrates.

"I stopped using drugs in treating my patients when I began to reexamine an old axiom, which is that nature is the true healer, using the body's natural defenses. The physician's role is to assist in that healing in cooperation with nature. Nature cures slowly just like trees grow slowly and not suddenly like chemical drug marketers claim. We tend to think of health as something that comes in a capsule purchased over the counter in a drugstore, instead of as a state which we attain by following the laws of nature."

- Dr. Henry G Bieler

Pears

Pears contain about 24% fiber and according to a study done reported in The 'American Journal of Epidemiology', fiber can actually improve lung function. After studying 15,792 men and women in London - aged 44 to 66 years with lung problems - scientists discovered that increasing dietary fiber actually reduces inflammation and improves lung function. They also discovered that other foods, such as processed foods, had detrimental effects on overall health.

Bronchitis	Kidneys
Cholesterol	Lungs
Colds	Menopause
Colon	Obesity
Constipation	Pain
Cramps	Parkinson's Disease
Digestion	Pneumonia
Diverticulitis	Rheumatism
Emphysema	Rosacea
Gall Stones	Shingles
Gallbladder	Sinus
Headache	Stroke
Hemorrhoids	Teeth/Gums
Hypoglycemia	Thyroid/Goiter
Inflammation	Ulcerative Colitis

One medium pear has 96 calories, no fat,
5 grams fiber, 26 grams carbohydrates.

Peas

Peas really can lower blood pressure. A study in at the University of Manitoba involved animals with polycystic disease, a severe form of kidney disease. Dr. Rotimi Aluko, the research scientist, fed small daily doses of pea protein (extracted from the yellow garden pea) to the animals. After eight weeks, he concluded that the animals had a 20 percent drop in blood pressure. "In people with high blood pressure, our protein could potentially delay or prevent the onset of kidney damage," said Rotimi Aluko, PhD. "In people who already have kidney disease, our protein may help them maintain normal blood pressure levels so they can live longer."

Allergies
Anemia
Blood Pressure
Bursitis
Cholesterol
Colds
Colon
Constipation
Cramps
Depression
Diverticulitis
Eyes
Heartburn
Hemorrhoids

Inflammation
Kidneys
Liver
Lungs
Lupus
Menopause
Multiple Sclerosis
Muscles/Ligaments
Nervousness
Obesity
Parkinson's Disease
Pneumonia
Premenstrual Syndrome
Rheumatism

Skin   Stroke

Stress   Thyroid/Goiter

One cup peas has 117 calories, 1 gram fat,
7 grams fiber, 21 grams carbohydrates.

Peppers (Sweet)

Peppers could actually help you lose weight. Researchers from the Exercise Metabolism Research Group, Department of Kinesiology at McMaster University in Ontario, studied the effects of capsinoids, the compounds found in sweet peppers, on twelve young men (average age 24). Half were given a placebo and the other half the capsinoid. Their findings were that the capsinoid group, after 90 minutes of moderately intense cycling, had much higher energy than the placebo group. They concluded that sweet peppers had potentially played a key role in the increased energy and certainly could be used as a weight loss aid.

Aging
Allergies
Alzheimer's Disease
Asthma
Atherosclerosis
Blood Pressure
Bronchitis
Circulation
Colds
Constipation
Diverticulitis
Energy
Eyes
Fingernails/Hair
Gout

Heart Disease
Hypoglycemia
Immune System
Influenza
Kidneys
Liver
Lungs
Menopause
Multiple Sclerosis
Obesity
Pain
Pancreas
Parkinson's Disease
Pneumonia
Premenstrual Syndrome

Prostate   Thyroid/Goiter

Sinus   Urinary Tract

Stress   Uterine Cancer

Stroke   Varicose Veins

Teeth/Gums

One medium sweet pepper has 23 calories, no fat,
2 grams fiber, 6 grams carbohydrates (+159% MDR vitamin C).

Persimmons

Persimmons with their high percentage of polyphenols may help you ward off a heart attack. Shela Gorinstein, Ph.D., who is a research associate with the Department of Medicinal Chemistry in the School of Pharmacy at the Hebrew University of Jerusalem in Israel, says that eating just one persimmon a day is enough to fight atherosclerosis. So maybe a persimmon a day keeps the doctor away.

Atherosclerosis   Lungs
Cholesterol   Multiple Sclerosis
Diarrhea   Rosacea
Heart Disease   Stroke
Influenza

One medium persimmon has 31 calories, no fat,
no fiber, 8 grams carbohydrates.

Pineapple

The pineapple, that wonderful fruit of Hawaii, may actually help with your joint pain. According to the University of Maryland Medical Center, the German Commission E has approved bromelain - the enzyme found in pineapple - after surgeries because it helps inflammation and swelling.

Arthritis/Joint Pain	Irritable Bowel Syndrome
Blood Pressure	Kidneys
Bronchitis	Lungs
Bursitis	Lupus
Circulation	Multiple Sclerosis
Colds	Muscles/Ligaments
Diarrhea	Obesity
Digestion	Osteoporosis
Diverticulitis	Pain
Emphysema	Pancreas
Eyes	Phlegm
Gas	Pneumonia
Gout	Rheumatism
Gum Disease	Shingles
Headache	Sinus
Heart Disease	Teeth/Gums
Heartburn	Thyroid/Goiter
Inflammation	Varicose Veins

One cup pineapple has 74 calories, no fat,
2 grams fiber, 20 grams carbohydrates.

Pomegranate

According to the April 2007 issue of 'Harvard Men's Health Watch', two studies on pomegranate juice indicated that it may be beneficial not only in fighting prostate cancer but in heart disease as well. Not only did pomegranate juice slow the rate of PSA increase, an important prostate cancer indicator, but it also protected LDL, the bad cholesterol from oxidative damage and it increased blood flow.

Aging
Alzheimer's Disease
Atherosclerosis
Breast Cancer
Cancer
Cholesterol
Circulation
Diabetes
Diarrhea
Gall Stones
Heart Disease
Hemorrhoids
Immune System

Inflammation
Lupus
Menopause
Muscles/Ligaments
Obesity
Prostate
Prostate Cancer
Rosacea
Skin
Skin Cancer
Teeth/Gums
Varicose Veins

One medium pomegranate has 104 calories, no fat,
1 gram fiber, 26 grams carbohydrates.

*"You can trace every sickness,
every disease and every ailment
to a mineral [a nutrient] deficiency."*

Dr. Linus Pauling, the only person in
history awarded two unshared Nobel Prizes.

Potatoes

Studies in Finland indicate the potatoes could reduce blood pressure. In the journal, 'Food Chemistry', researchers from MTT Agrifood Research found that the ACE inhibitor and anti-oxidants in potatoes are the reasons. Lead author Anne Pihlanto stated, "The results of this study suggest that potato is a promising source for the production of bioactive compounds as ingredients for developing functional foods with a beneficial impact on cardiovascular health."

Allergies	Insomnia
Alzheimer's Disease	Liver
Atherosclerosis	Multiple Sclerosis
Blood Pressure	Muscles/Ligaments
Constipation	Nervousness
Cramps	Pain
Depression	Pancreas
Diarrhea	Parkinson's Disease
Diverticulitis	Pneumonia
Emphysema	Premenstrual Syndrome
Energy	Prostate
Gout	Rheumatism
Headache	Shingles
Heart Disease	Stress
Heartburn	Ulcerative Colitis
Hemorrhoids	Urinary Tract
Hepatitis	

One medium potato has 164 calories, no fat,
5 grams fiber, 37 grams carbohydrates.

Prunes

Concerned about low bone density? Have some prunes. According to researchers from the University of Oklahoma Health Sciences and Oklahoma State University, the reason is the polyphenols. The study, reported in the 'Journal of Nutritional Biochemistry', stated that,"It is possible that dietary consumption of dried (prunes) could serve as a source of polyphenolic compounds that favourably modulate both bone formation and resorption, and provide a natural alternative for individuals at risk of osteoporosis."

Aging
Alzheimer's Disease
Anemia
Blood Pressure
Cholesterol
Circulation
Colon
Constipation
Cramps
Depression
Diverticulitis

Gall Stones
Gallbladder
Heart Disease
Hemorrhoids
Irritable Bowel Syndrome
Menopause
Nervousness
Osteoporosis
Rosacea
Stroke

One medium prune has 19 calories, no fat,
1 gram fiber, 5 grams carbohydrates.

Pumpkin/Pumpkin Seeds

According to the scientists at Harvard School of Public Health, pumpkin can lower the risk of lung cancer. This is due to the huge antioxidant protection of beta-cryptoxanthin, a carotenoid present in pumpkin. Another health benefit is that it is also important for your eyes because of a second carotenoid, beta-carotene, that converts vitamin A in the body. A recent study showed that people whose intake of vitamin A was highest had a 43% lower risk of developing age-related macular degeneration.

Acne
Alzheimer's Disease
Anemia
Arthritis/Joint Pain
Bronchitis
Bursitis
Cancer
Cervical Cancer
Cholesterol
Circulation
Colds
Constipation
Depression
Diabetes
Eyes
Fibromyalgia

Fingernails/Hair
Gas
Gout
Heart Disease
Hemorrhoids
Immune System
Inflammation
Influenza
Insomnia
Irritable Bowel Syndrome
Lung Cancer
Lungs
Lupus
Multiple Sclerosis
Muscles/Ligaments
Obesity

Osteoporosis

Pain

Pneumonia

Premenstrual Syndrome

Prostate

Rosacea

Shingles

Sinus

Thyroid/Goiter

Ulcers

One cup pumpkin seeds has 30 calories, no fat,
1 gram fiber, 8 grams carbohydrates.

One ounce (142 pumpkin seeds) has 151 calories,
13 grams fat, 1 gram fiber, 5 grams carbohydrates.

Raisins

The University of Maine presented a study to the 2001 Experimental Biology conference in Orlando, Florida that the dietary fiber and other components in raisins may reduce the risk of both heart disease and cancer, due to the fact that raisins bind bile acids in the intestine and cause them to be excreted. Without this binding, bile acids might turn into molecules that could enhance cancer growth. This binding had a second benefit – it lowers cholesterol which reduces the risk of heart disease.

Anemia	Gall Stones
Arthritis/Joint Pain	Heart Disease
Blood Pressure	Hemorrhoids
Cancer	Influenza
Cholesterol	Multiple Sclerosis
Constipation	Obesity
Cramps	Osteoporosis
Digestion	Pain
Energy	Thyroid/Goiter
Eyes	Ulcers

One cup raisins has 493 calories, 1 gram fat,
6 grams fiber, 131 grams carbohydrates.

Raspberries

Raspberries, rich in resveratrol, may be the weapon you need against Alzheimer's disease, dementia and memory loss. According to research conducted in the Netherlands the antioxidant in raspberries is exceptionally high. In fact, it is 50% higher than strawberries, up to three times higher than kiwi, and ten times higher than lycopene-rich tomatoes.

Aging
Allergies
Alzheimer's Disease
Arthritis/Joint Pain
Asthma
Bronchitis
Colds
Constipation
Diabetes
Digestion
Emphysema
Energy
Esophageal Cancer
Eyes
Gall Stones
Gallbladder
Hepatitis
Hypoglycemia
Immune System

Inflammation
Irritable Bowel Syndrome
Kidneys
Liver
Lupus
Menopause
Muscles/Ligaments
Nervousness
Obesity
Pain
Pancreas
Parkinson's Disease
Phlegm
Premenstrual Syndrome
Prostate
Rheumatism
Sinus
Stress
Thyroid/Goiter

Ulcerative Colitis   Uterine Cancer

Ulcers   Varicose Veins

One cup raspberries has 63 calories, 1 gram fat,
8 grams fiber, 15 grams carbohydrates.

"If we doctors threw all our medicines into the sea, it would be that much better for our patients and that much worse for the fishes."

—Supreme Court Justice Oliver Wendell Holmes, MD

Sesame Seeds

Sesame seeds could reduce the risk of heart disease. A study published in the 'Journal of Food Science' stated that when a protein isolate that comes from sesame seeds was fed to animals on a high cholesterol diet, their (bad) LDL levels were lowered and their (good) HDL levels increased by a whopping 41%.

Anemia

Cholesterol

Fibromyalgia

Heart Disease

Hemorrhoids

Insomnia

Liver

Lupus

Nervousness

Obesity

Osteoporosis

Parkinson's Disease

Pneumonia

Teeth/Gums

Thyroid/Goiter

One tablespoon sesame seeds has 51 calories, 4 grams fat,
1 gram fiber, 2 grams carbohydrates.

*"Life expectancy would grow by leaps and bounds
if green vegetables smelled as good as bacon."*

—Doug Larson

Spinach

Concerned about that memory of yours slipping? Have some spinach. In a controlled animal study at the USDA Human Nutrition Research Center on Aging at Tufts University in Boston, researchers discovered that spinach helped to diminish brain function problems and helped in disorders like Alzheimer's and Parkinson's disease. Just a daily dose of spinach not only helped protect nerve cells from the effects of aging, but contributed to a better long term memory.

Acne	Cramps
Aging	Depression
Allergies	Diabetes
Alzheimer's Disease	Digestion
Anemia	Emphysema
Arthritis/Joint Pain	Energy
Asthma	Eyes
Atherosclerosis	Fibromyalgia
Blood Pressure	Fingernails/Hair
Breast Cancer	Gall Stones
Bronchitis	Gas
Cancer	Headache
Cervical Cancer	Heart Disease
Circulation	Hemorrhoids
Colds	Hepatitis
Colon	Hypoglycemia
Colon Cancer	Immune System
Constipation	Inflammation

Insomnia

Irritable Bowel Syndrome

Liver

Lung Cancer

Lungs

Lupus

Menopause

Multiple Sclerosis

Muscles/Ligaments

Nervousness

Obesity

Osteoporosis

Pain

Pancreas

Parkinson's Disease

Phlegm

Pneumonia

Premenstrual Syndrome

Prostate

Rosacea

Shingles

Sinus

Skin

Stress

Stroke

Teeth/Gums

Thyroid/Goiter

Ulcers

Urinary Tract

Varicose Veins

One cup spinach has 6 calories, no fat,
1 gram fiber, 1 gram carbohydrates.

Squash

Squash is a powerhouse in the fight against cancer. The National Cancer Institute says that squash is one of the top three foods for the prevention and control of lung cancer. A recent study found that smokers who ate 2 ½ servings of squash a day greatly risked their risk of lung cancer. The Tokyo National Cancer Institute backs up the cancer fighting ability of squash and adds that winter squash is at the top of the vegetable list as a factor in populations with low cancer rates.

Acne	Emphysema
Alzheimer's Disease	Eyes
Anemia	Fibromyalgia
Arthritis/Joint Pain	Fingernails/Hair
Asthma	Headache
Atherosclerosis	Heart Disease
Blood Pressure	Hemorrhoids
Bronchitis	Hepatitis
Cancer	Hypoglycemia
Colds	Immune System
Colon	Inflammation
Colon Cancer	Insomnia
Constipation	Irritable Bowel Syndrome
Cramps	Kidneys
Diabetes	Liver
Diarrhea	Lung Cancer

Lungs

Lupus

Menopause

Multiple Sclerosis

Muscles/Ligaments

Nervousness

Obesity

Osteoporosis

Pain

Pancreas

Parkinson's Disease

Premenstrual Syndrome

Prostate

Prostate Cancer

Rheumatism

Rosacea

Shingles

Thyroid/Goiter

Ulcerative Colitis

Urinary Tract

Uterine Cancer

One cup summer squash has 18 calories, no fat,
1 gram fiber, 4 grams carbohydrates.

One cup winter squash has 39 calories, no fat,
2 grams fiber, 10 grams carbohydrates.

Strawberries

Researchers have found that strawberries, especially organic strawberries, are a powerful force against cancer cells. At a lab study at the Swedish University of Agricultural Sciences, a study was done on human colon and breast cancer cells using strawberry extracts. At the highest concentration, the non organic extracts killed 49% of the colon cancer cells and 37.9% of the breast cancer cells. When they used the organic extracts, 60% of the colon cancer cells and 53.1% of the breast cancer cells were killed.

Acne	Cramps
Aging	Depression
Allergies	Diabetes
Alzheimer's Disease	Digestion
Arthritis/Joint Pain	Eyes
Asthma	Gall Stones
Atherosclerosis	Gallbladder
Blood Pressure	Gout
Breast Cancer	Heart Disease
Bronchitis	Hepatitis
Bursitis	Hypoglycemia
Cancer	Immune System
Circulation	Inflammation
Colds	Influenza
Colon	Insomnia
Colon Cancer	Irritable Bowel Syndrome
Constipation	Kidneys

Liver	Prostate
Lungs	Rheumatism
Lupus	Shingles
Menopause	Sinus
Multiple Sclerosis	Skin
Muscles/Ligaments	Stress
Nervousness	Stroke
Obesity	Ulcerative Colitis
Pain	Uterine Cancer
Parkinson's Disease	Varicose Veins

One cup strawberries has 46 calories, no fat,
3 grams fiber, 11 grams carbohydrates (+141% MDR vitamin C).

When diet is wrong, medicine is of no use.
When diet is correct, medicine is of no need.

—Ancient Ayurvedic Proverb

Sunflower Seeds

Research has shown that sunflower seed oil may be useful in fighting multiple sclerosis. The 'British Medical Journal' reported that scientists at the Royal Victoria Hospital in Belfast, Northern Ireland led a test group of seventy-five patients who all had multiple sclerosis. The group was split into two groups – one being given two tablespoons of sunflower seed oil a day and the other one being given two tablespoons of olive oil. At the end of the study the lead doctor, Dr. Harold Millar, concluded that the group who had taken the sunflower oil showed significant improvement.

Allergies

Anemia

Arthritis/Joint Pain

Blood Pressure

Cholesterol

Circulation

Colon

Constipation

Cramps

Depression

Digestion

Eyes

Fibromyalgia

Heart Disease

Hemorrhoids

Inflammation

Insomnia

Irritable Bowel Syndrome

Multiple Sclerosis

Muscles/Ligaments

Premenstrual Syndrome
(unsalted sunflower seeds)

Prostate

Radiation Exposure

Stress

Stroke

Thyroid/Goiter

Ulcers

One cup sunflower seeds has 820 calories,
71 grams fat (7 grams saturated),
15 grams fiber, 27 grams carbohydrates.

Sweet Potatoes

Interested in reducing your risk of stroke, heart disease and cancer? Follow the Japanese diet. The people of Okinawa, Japan have the longest disability-free life expectancy in the world. They are physically active, do not smoke and eat a diet high in vegetables – and sweet potatoes are a prominent part of their diet. Many physicians including Dr. Robert Cornell, emeritus professor of cardiothoracic surgery of Wake Forest University School of Medicine highly recommend them. He recently said, "Sweet potatoes contain significant deterrents to heart disease and stroke. In addition, reports have suggested anti-cancer effects. With these facts in mind, all of us should make sweet potatoes a more frequent part of our regular diet." The North Carolina Stroke Association, the American Cancer Society and the American Heart Association agree and have all endorsed sweet potatoes as a nutritious food that is helpful in the prevention of disease.

Alzheimer's Disease

Anemia

Arthritis/Joint Pain

Blood Pressure

Breast Cancer

Bronchitis

Cancer

Circulation

Colds

Colon

Colon Cancer

Constipation

Diabetes

Digestion

Diverticulitis

Emphysema

Eyes

Fibromyalgia

Fingernails/Hair

Gall Stones

Gallbladder

Headache

Heart Disease

Hemorrhoids

Hepatitis

Immune System

Inflammation

Influenza

Irritable Bowel Syndrome

Liver

Lungs

Lupus

Menopause

Multiple Sclerosis

Muscles/Ligaments

Nervousness

Obesity

Osteoporosis

Pain

Pancreas

Parkinson's Disease

Pneumonia

Premenstrual Syndrome

Prostate

Rectal Cancer

Rheumatism

Rosacea

Shingles

Skin Cancer

Stomach Cancer

Stress

Stroke

Thyroid/Goiter

Ulcerative Colitis

Ulcers

Urinary Tract

Varicose Veins

One cup sweet potatoes has 114 calories, no fat,
4 grams fiber, 27 grams carbohydrates (+377% MDR vitamin A).

Swiss Chard

The Framingham Heart Study found that people who consumed 250 mcg of vitamin K a day had a 35% lower risk of hip fractures compared to those who consumed less. The good news is that it's easy to protect your bone health with vitamin K rich foods like Swiss chard. Just ½ cup cooked Swiss chard provides 88g – over 350% of the daily recommended value.

Aging

Alzheimer's Disease

Anemia

Bronchitis

Bursitis

Constipation

Cramps

Diabetes

Diverticulitis

Energy

Esophageal Cancer

Fibromyalgia

Fingernails/Hair

Gallbladder

Gas

Headache

Hypoglycemia

Inflammation

Irritable Bowel Syndrome

Lungs

Lupus

Menopause

Multiple Sclerosis

Muscles/Ligaments

Osteoporosis

Pain

Pancreas

Parkinson's Disease

Phlegm

Premenstrual Syndrome

Prostate

Rosacea

Shingles

Stress

Stroke

Ulcers

One cup swiss chard has 6 calories, no fat,
1 gram fiber, 1 gram carbohydrates.

"It's supposed to be a secret, but I'll tell you anyway. We doctors do nothing. We only help and encourage the doctor within."

—Albert Schweitzer, M.D.

Tomatoes

According to a meta-analysis of 21 studies which was published in 'Cancer Epidemiology Biomarkers and Prevention', men who consumed the highest of amount of raw tomatoes had an 11% reduction of risk for prostate cancer and those who consumed cooked tomatoes were found to have a 19% reduction in risk. It stems from the synergy between the photonutrients and lycopene naturally present in tomatoes.

Acne	Cramps
Aging	Diabetes
Allergies	Emphysema
Alzheimer's Disease	Eyes
Anemia	Gall Stones
Atherosclerosis	Gallbladder
Blood Pressure	Gout
Breast Cancer	Headache
Bronchitis	Heart Disease
Cancer	Hepatitis
Cervical Cancer	Hypoglycemia
Cholesterol	Immune System
Circulation	Inflammation
Colds	Influenza
Colon	Liver
Colon Cancer	Lungs
Constipation	Menopause

Multiple Sclerosis

Muscles/Ligaments

Obesity

Osteoporosis

Pancreas

Parkinson's Disease

Phlegm

Premenstrual Syndrome

Prostate

Prostate Cancer

Rheumatism

Shingles

Sinus

Skin Cancer

Stomach Cancer

Stress

Teeth/Gums

Thyroid/Goiter

Ulcerative Colitis

Ulcers

Urinary Tract

Uterine Cancer

One medium tomato has 22 calories, no fat,
1 gram fiber, 5 grams carbohydrates.

Turnips

Feeling a little down lately? Maybe even confused? It could be due to a nutritional deficiency in your system. A study in the July, 2004 issue of the American Journal of Clinical Nutrition, reported that when 228 subjects were evaluated, it was found that of those whose bloods levels of folate were the lowest, their risk of mild cognitive impairment more than tripled. So protect yourself by adding some folate rich food to your diet. One of the foods highest in folate is turnip greens. Just one cup provides 170 mcg.

Acne

Aging (especially turnip greens)

Anemia

Asthma (especially turnip greens)

Blood Pressure (especially turnip greens)

Bronchitis (especially turnip greens)

Bursitis

Colds (especially turnip greens)

Colon

Constipation (especially greens)

Depression

Digestion

Diverticulitis

Gout (especially turnip greens)

Immune System (especially turnip greens)

Inflammation

Insomnia (especially turnip greens)

Irritable Bowel Syndrome

Kidneys

Liver (especially turnip greens)

Lungs

Menopause

Multiple Sclerosis

Muscles/Ligaments

Obesity

Osteoporosis (especially turnip greens)

Pain

Pneumonia   Shingles

Rosacea   Teeth/Gums

One medium turnip has 34 calories, no fat,
2 grams fiber, 8 grams carbohydrates.

Walnuts

The results from a recent lab study at the University of California at Davis found that walnuts can actually slow the growth of prostate tumors. In the 18 week trial, half of the animals with prostate cancer tumors were fed ground up walnuts – the other half were fed a diet high in fat from soybean oil. At the end of the study, the animals on the walnut diet exhibited not only reductions of tumor growth but also it was evident in their bloodstream. So how many walnuts would be equal to what the animals were fed? About 500 calories or ¾ cup a day.

Aging
Alzheimer's Disease
Anemia
Arthritis/Joint Pain
Asthma
Atherosclerosis
Blood Pressure
Bronchitis
Cancer
Cholesterol
Circulation
Colon
Colon Cancer
Depression
Diabetes

Digestion
Energy
Eyes
Fibromyalgia
Fingernails/Hair
Gall Stones
Heart Disease
Hepatitis
Immune System
Inflammation
Kidneys
Lungs
Menopause
Multiple Sclerosis
Muscles/Ligaments

Nervousness	Sinus
Obesity	Skin
Osteoporosis	Skin Cancer
Parkinson's Disease	Stroke
Premenstrual Syndrome	Teeth/Gums
Prostate Cancer	Thyroid/Goiter
Rheumatism	

One cup walnuts has 654 calories, 65 grams fat, 7 grams fiber, 14 grams carbohydrates.

"One of the biggest tragedies of human civilization is the precedent of chemical therapy over nutrition. It's a substitution of artificial therapy over nature, of poisons over food, in which we are feeding people poisons trying to correct the reactions of starvation."

—Dr. Royal Lee, January 12, 1951

Watercress

Can watercress suppress breast cancer cell development? The University of Southhampton thinks so. This study was published in both the 'Bristish Journal of Nutrition' and in 'Biochemical Pharmacology'. The researchers did a pilot study of breast cancer survivors who underwent a period of fasting before eating 80g. (about a cereal bowl full) of watercress. Over the next 24 hours blood samples were taken and they discovered that the compounds in the watercress were able to interfere with proteins that cause cancer development.

Aging
Alzheimer's Disease
Blood Pressure
Breast Cancer
Cancer
Cholesterol
Circulation
Colds
Headache
Influenza
Irritable Bowel Syndrome
Kidney Stones
Kidneys
Lungs
Multiple Sclerosis
Muscles/Ligaments
Obesity
Phlegm
Premenstrual Syndrome
Shingles
Thyroid/Goiter

One cup watercress has 3 calories, no fat,
no fiber, no carbohydrates.

Watermelon

Is your blood pressure creeping up? Have some watermelon. Florida State University recently did a study on nine middle-aged prehypertension patients. Scientists gave the participants six grams of watermelon extract a day for six weeks. At the end of the study all nine patients had lowered blood pressure. The researchers concluded that these findings suggest that watermelon may prevent prehypertension from turning into full-blown hypertension – a major risk for heart attacks and stroke.

Anemia	Obesity
Blood Pressure	Parkinson's Disease
Cancer	Phlegm
Cholesterol	Prostate
Circulation	Rosacea
Gall Stones	Shingles
Heart Disease	Skin
Influenza	Stroke
Irritable Bowel Syndrome	Teeth/Gums
Kidneys	Thyroid/Goiter
Lungs	

One cup watermelon has 45 calories, no fat,
1 gram fiber, 11 grams carbohydrates.

Wheat Germ

The University of Maryland Medical Center states that wheat germ as been shown to slow the progression of Alzheimer's disease. The Omega-3 fatty acids found in wheat germ are important for brain memory and performance.

Alzheimer's Disease
Atherosclerosis
Blood Pressure
Breast Cancer
Cancer
Cholesterol
Circulation
Colon
Colon Cancer
Constipation
Depression
Diabetes
Digestion
Diverticulitis
Energy
Esophageal Cancer
Eyes
Fingernails/Hair
Gall Stones
Gas
Headache

Heart Disease
Heartburn
Hemorrhoids
Hepatitis
Liver
Menopause
Muscles/Ligaments
Nervousness
Obesity
Osteoporosis
Parkinson's Disease
Premenstrual Syndrome
Prostate
Rosacea
Skin
Stomach Cancer
Stress
Stroke
Thyroid/Goiter
Varicose Veins

One cup wheat germ has 413 calories, 11 grams fat,
15 grams fiber, 60 grams carbohydrates.

Yogurt

Does low-fat yogurt really help you lose weight? The University of Tennessee says it does. They did a 12 week study of 34 obese, but otherwise healthy, adults and divided them into two groups. The first group consumed low fat yogurt three times a day (1100 mg of calcium a day). The second group consumed a low calcium diet with only one serving of calcium each day. At the end of the study the yogurt group lost 22% more weight (an average of 14 pounds), 66% more body fat and 81% more trunkal (stomach) fat.

Aging	Diverticulitis
Allergies	Eyes
Alzheimer's Disease	Fibromyalgia
Asthma	Fingernails/Hair
Blood Pressure	Gall Stones
Bronchitis	Gas
Cancer	Gout
Cholesterol	Hepatitis
Circulation	Heart Disease
Colds	Hypoglycemia
Colon	Immune System
Colon Cancer	Inflammation
Constipation	Influenza
Cramps	Insomnia
Diarrhea	Irritable Bowel Syndrome
Digestion	Liver

Lupus   Premenstrual Syndrome
Menopause   Shingles
Multiple Sclerosis   Sinus
Muscles/Ligaments   Skin
Nausea   Stress
Nervousness   Teeth/Gums
Obesity   Ulcerative Colitis
Osteoporosis   Ulcers
Pain   Urinary Tract
Pancreas   Uterine Cancer
Parkinson's Disease

One cup low-fat yogurt has 154 calories, 4 grams fat,
no fiber, 17 grams carbohydrates.

"We must admit that we have never fought the homeopath on matters of principle. We fought them because they came into our community and got the business."

—Dr. J.N. McCormack, AMA, 1903

Part II

Helpful Herbs and Spices

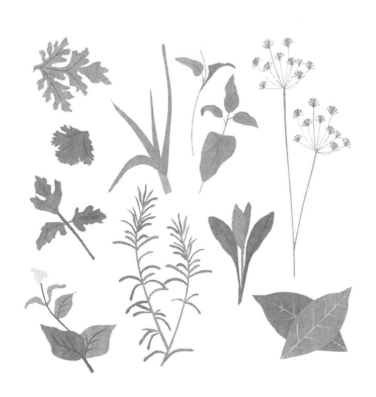

The World Health Organization (WHO) states that in Asian and African countries, 80% of the population depend on traditional herbal medicine. Additionally, the use of herbs in the United States has expanded significantly in the past decade. Herbs are indeed powerful medicine, and as such, precautions must be taken. Always check with your physician to be certain that there is no interaction with your prescribed medicines.

Alfalfa

In the first human study on alfalfa, Indiana University School of Medicine determined that alfalfa substantially reduced cholesterol. The patients entered the study with over 50% taking statin drugs (Mevacor, Lipitor, Zocor) and over 60% suffering from coronary artery disease. The patients were divided into three groups. The first group was on a placebo pill, the second group was given 1120 mg. of alfalfa day and the third group was given 2240 mg of alfalfa a day. After six weeks, the groups were compared. As expected, no change in the placebo group, but the level of (LDL) bad cholesterol in the alfalfa groups declined and average of 16.6% and the level of (HDL) good cholesterol increased an average of 11.2%. It was also noted that the inflammation in the blood (C-reactive protein) was significantly reduced – 24% reduction in the 1120 mg. group, but a huge 50.4% in the group taking the most alfalfa.

Acne	Diverticulitis
Allergies	Energy
Anemia	Fingernails/Hair
Arthritis/Joint Pain	Gallbladder
Bursitis	Gout
Cholesterol	Heart Disease
Colon	Inflammation
Colon Cancer	Irritable Bowel Syndrome
Constipation	Kidneys
Cramps	Liver
Diabetes	Lungs
Digestion	Lupus

Multiple Sclerosis

Sinus

Nausea

Skin

Obesity

Teeth/Gums

Osteoporosis

Ulcerative Colitis

Rheumatism

Ulcers

Rosacea

Shingles

Aloe Vera

The famous cancer research clinic in Houston, M.D. Anderson, found that aloe vera protects the immune cells in the skin. They further stated that the adverse effects of sun exposure are neutralized with aloe vera and that even previous damage can be reversed resulting in younger-looking healthier skin.

Acne

Aging

Burns

Colon

Colon Cancer

Constipation

Digestion

Diverticulitis

Emphysema

Heartburn

Hemorrhoids

Immune System

Inflammation

Irritable Bowel Syndrome

Liver

Lungs

Lupus

Menopause

Obesity

Rosacea

Shingles

Skin

Skin Cancer

Teeth/Gums

Ulcerative Colitis

Ulcers

Varicose Veins

"We tend to think of health as something that comes in a capsule purchased over the counter in a drugstore, instead of as a state which we attain by following the laws of nature."

— Dr. Henry G Bieler, M.D.

Basil

According to a study presented at the British Pharmaceutical Conference in Manchester, England, basil can help relieve arthritis. Basil compounds were given to arthritic patients and in just 24 hours, arthritic swelling was reduced a remarkable 73%. They found that the compounds in basil (eugenol and ursolic) , not only relieve swelling but relieve pain as well.

Aging	Eyes
Allergies	Gas
Arthritis/Joint Pain	Headache
Asthma	Heart Disease
Atherosclerosis	Inflammation
Bronchitis	Influenza
Cholesterol	Liver
Circulation	Nausea
Colds	Nervousness
Constipation	Pain
Cramps	Rosacea
Depression	Sinus
Digestion	Stress
Emphysema	

Bee Pollen

Researchers from the Department of Urology at the University of Wales recently performed a double blind study on 60 men with prostate enlargement. Half were given a placebo, and the other half were given bee pollen extract. The results determined that those who received the bee pollen showed a 69% improvement – and no side effects.

Aging

Allergies

Alzheimer's Disease

Asthma

Cancer

Digestion

Energy

Hypoglycemia

Immune System

Lupus

Obesity

Prostate

Stress

Cardamom

Cardamom is not only a wonderful spice to add to recipes, like Finnish bread, but it also packs a powerful punch against high blood pressure. A study for the Drug Research Center at RNT Medical College in India found that oral consumption of 3g of cardamom a day for 12 weeks significantly lowered systolic, diastolic and mean blood pressure in newly diagnosed patients with hypertension.

Allergies	Gas
Asthma	Liver
Blood Pressure	Lungs
Bronchitis	Nausea
Circulation	Obesity
Cramps	Sinus
Digestion	Urinary Tract
Energy	

Cayenne Pepper

You might think that spicy food would increase blood pressure, but in fact it does just the opposite. In 2010, a study was published in the journal, 'Cell Metabolism', stating that researchers at the University of North Carolina discovered that capsaicin (cayenne) increased nitric oxide in the body. This gas actually dilates blood vessels, which improves blood pressure.

Acne
Alzheimer's Disease
Arthritis/Joint Pain
Asthma
Atherosclerosis
Blood Pressure (high)
Bronchitis
Circulation
Colds
Cramps
Diabetes
Diarrhea
Digestion
Energy
Eyes
Gas
Headache
Heart Disease
Heartburn
Hemorrhoids
Immune System

Inflammation
Influenza
Irritable Bowel Syndrome
Kidneys
Liver
Lungs
Muscles/Ligaments
Obesity
Phlegm
Pneumonia
Premenstrual Syndrome
Rheumatism
Shingles
Sinus
Stress
Teeth/Gums
Ulcerative Colitis
Ulcers
Varicose Veins

Chamomile

Chamomile has long been known to relieve stress, but it was actually proven on a study done by the University of Pennsylvania. In a double-blind 8 week trial, participants were divided into two groups. One group received a placebo and the other received a 220mg chamomile capsule daily. Doses were adjusted up to five capsules a day and researchers used the Hamilton Anxiety Rating to measure results. At the end of the study, the chamomile patients had a significant reduction in anxiety over the placebo group.

Asthma
Colds
Cramps
Digestion
Diverticulitis
Eyes
Gas
Headache
Hemorrhoids
Hepatitis
Immune System
Inflammation
Insomnia
Irritable Bowel Syndrome

Kidneys
Liver
Nausea
Nervousness
Pain
Premenstrual Syndrome
Rosacea
Shingles
Stress
Teeth/Gums
Ulcerative Colitis
Varicose Veins

"A cure that grows in the backyard is not going to increase anyone's dividends."

— Lehane, The Power of Plants, 1977

Chili Pepper

Chili peppers can not only help with diabetes but also with your weight according to an article published in the 'American Journal of Clinical Nutrition'. A study at the University of Tasmania found that the normal eating of chili peppers can significantly control insulin levels. Their study was able to prove that after eating chilies, the body's blood sugar lowered by an incredible 60%.

Allergies
Arthritis/Joint Pain
Asthma
Blood Pressure (high)
Cancer
Cholesterol
Circulation
Colds
Depression
Diabetes
Digestion
Emphysema
Fibromyalgia
Heart Disease
Hepatitis

Immune System
Inflammation
Influenza
Insomnia
Obesity
Pain
Phlegm
Shingles
Sinus
Skin Cancer
Stroke
Ulcers

Cinnamon

Researchers at the U.S. Department of Agriculture in Beltsville, Maryland, have found that cinnamon increases three important proteins in your body that promotes normal insulin-signaling processes helping to stabilize diabetes. Scientists at the University of Sweden confirmed these findings with a study of their own involving 14 healthy people. Using ultrasound imaging, they monitored the GER (gastric emptying rata) after the study group ate two bowls of rice pudding – one without cinnamon and the other with cinnamon. They found that those who ate the cinnamon spiced pudding had a drastically delayed GER which lowered their blood sugar levels. Post-meal blood sugar (glucose) levels have been linked to a higher risk of diabetes complications such as heart disease.

Alzheimer's Disease	Heartburn
Arthritis/Joint Pain	Immune System
Cholesterol	Inflammation
Circulation	Irritable Bowel Syndrome
Colds	Menopause
Colon Cancer	Nausea
Diabetes	Obesity
Diarrhea	Pancreas
Digestion	Premenstrual Syndrome
Gas	Teeth/Gums
Headache	
Heart Disease	

Cloves

A double-blind study was done at the U.S. Department of Agriculture in Beltsville, Maryland on the connection between cloves and levels of glucose and cholesterol in the body. They discovered that the patients who ingested cloves, regardless of the amount of cloves consumed, showed a drop in levels of glucose, triglycerides and LDL (bad) cholesterol. Blood levels of HDL (good) cholesterol were not affected among the clove eaters and most significantly, those who did not ingest cloves experienced no change.

Acne

Aging

Breast Cancer

Cancer

Cholesterol

Colds

Cramps

Dental

Depression

Diabetes

Digestion

Diverticulitis

Gas

Hepatitis

Immune System

Inflammation

Influenza

Kidneys

Liver

Lupus

Multiple Sclerosis

Nausea

Obesity

Pancreas

Parkinson's Disease

Prostate

Prostate Cancer

Shingles

Sinus

Skin

Teeth/Gums

Ulcerative Colitis

"You cannot poison your body into health with drugs, chemo or radiation. Health can only be achieved with healthful living."

—T.C. Fry

Dandelion

Dandelion is a natural diuretic and has been known to increase urine to cleanse the kidneys. The University of Maryland Medical Center has stated that some preliminary tests have shown that dandelion may help to normalize blood pressure. In Europe dandelion has been long known for its medicinal properties. In fact, the German Commission E (similar to the US FDA) recommends dandelion for treatment in liver disorders and digestion.

Acne

Aging

Allergies

Alzheimer's Disease

Anemia

Atherosclerosis

Blood Pressure (low)

Breast Cancer

Bronchitis

Cancer

Circulation

Constipation

Cramps

Diabetes

Digestion

Emphysema

Energy

Fibromyalgia

Fingernails/Hair

Gall Stones

Gallbladder

Gout

Heartburn

Hepatitis

Immune Disease

Influenza

Insomnia

Irritable Bowel Syndrome

Kidneys

Liver

Menopause

Multiple Sclerosis

Muscles/Ligaments

Obesity

Osteoporosis

Pancreas

Parkinson's Disease

Premenstrual Syndrome

Prostate Cancer

Radiation exposure

Rosacea

Shingles

Sinus

Skin

Ulcerative Colitis

Varicose Veins

Echinacea

Germany's Commission E has approved Echinacea for treating respiratory infections and urinary tract infections. In a study from the University of Connecticut, researchers found that Echinacea can be helpful in shortening the duration of a cold by 1.4 days. They further stated that taking Echinacea alone was found to reduce the risk of catching a cold by 58% but taking a combination of vitamin C and Echinacea reduced the risk of cold incidence by a whopping 86%.

Acne

Aging

Asthma

Blood Purifier

Breast Cancer

Bronchitis

Cancer

Colds

Immune System

Inflammation

Influenza

Liver

Pancreas

Parkinson's Disease

Phlegm

Pneumonia

Prostate

Prostate Cancer

Shingles

Teeth/Gums

Urinary Tract

"Garlics, tho' used by the French, are better adapted to the uses of medicine than cookery."

— Amelia Simmons, 'American Cookery' (1796)

Garlic

Garlic is a natural antibiotic and has been called "Russian penicillin" because of its ability to fight disease and infection and even lower blood pressure. At the Clinical Research Center in New Orleans, Louisiana, an open study was done on the effect garlic has on blood pressure. Nine patients with severe hypertension were given 2400 mg of allicin, a compound in garlic. The results were impressive. Sitting blood pressure was lowered just five hours after taking the garlic and continued to stabilize for several hours with no side effects reported.

Garlic has also been effectively used against MRSA (a staph infection that is responsible for over 350,000 people being hospitalized each year and over 19,000 deaths in the U.S. alone every year.) The World Health Organization calls MRSA the most important health issue of the 21st century. Unlike prescription drugs that become ineffective after a period of time and weaken your system, garlic boosts your immune system and has been clinically proven at the University of East London to effectively cure MRSA in just 4 to 12 weeks.

Acne	Breast Cancer
Aging	Bronchitis
Allergies	Cancer
Alzheimer's Disease	Cholesterol
Arthritis/Joint Pain	Circulation
Asthma	Colds
Atherosclerosis	Colon Cancer
Blood Pressure (high)	Cramps

Depression

Diarrhea

Digestion

Diverticulitis

Emphysema

Eyes

Fibromyalgia

Gall Stones

Gallbladder

Headache

Heart Disease

Hemorrhoids

Hepatitis

Immune System

Inflammation

Influenza

Kidneys

Liver

Lungs

Lupus

Multiple Sclerosis

Muscles/Ligaments

Obesity

Osteoporosis

Pain

Pancreas

Parkinson's Disease

Phlegm

Pneumonia

Premenstrual Syndrome

Prostate

Prostate Cancer

Rheumatism

Shingles

Sinus

Stomach Cancer

Stroke

Ulcers

Varicose Veins

Ginger

Ginger has long been known to help nausea and control inflammation, but the University of Michigan Comprehensive Cancer Center is now investigating ginger as a treatment for ovarian cancer. In laboratory studies, researchers used ginger powder, similar to that sold in grocery stores, which they dissolved and applied to ovarian cancer cells. The results were consistent. The ginger solution killed all of the ovarian cancer cells tested.

Aging	Gall Stones
Allergies	Gallbladder
Arthritis/Joint Pain	Gas
Atherosclerosis	Gout
Breast Cancer	Headache
Bronchitis	Heart Disease
Cancer	Heartburn
Cholesterol	Hemorrhoids
Circulation	Hepatitis
Colds	Immune System
Colon	Inflammation
Colon Cancer	Influenza
Cramps	Insomnia
Depression	Irritable Bowel Syndrome
Diarrhea	Liver
Digestion	Lungs
Emphysema	Nausea
Fibromyalgia	Nervousness

Obesity

Ovarian Cancer

Pain

Pancreas

Phlegm

Pneumonia

Premenstrual Syndrome

Rheumatism

Radiation exposure

Rosacea

Shingles

Sinus

Skin

Stress

Stroke

Stomach Cancer

Teeth/Gums

Ulcerative Colitis

Ulcers

Varicose Veins

Ginkgo Biloba

Mayo Clinic has stated that there is promising evidence favoring the use of ginkgo biloba to enhance memory as a help to fighting diseases like Alzheimer's. In 2006 the Brain Research Institute at UCLA did a double-blind study determining the use of ginkgo biloba and memory impairment. The study involved 10 patients, aged 45 to 75, who did not have dementia but complained of memory loss. Four of the patients received 120 mg of ginkgo biloba a day and the other six received a placebo. At the end of six months, the scientists determined that there was significant improvement in verbal recall among those who were given ginkgo biloba. They stated the gingko biloba patients had better brain function in key brain memory centers.

Aging	Heart Disease
Allergies	Immune System
Alzheimer's Disease	Kidneys
Asthma	Multiple Sclerosis
Breast Cancer	Nervousness
Bronchitis	Parkinson's Disease
Circulation	Radiation exposure
Cramps	Sinus
Depression	Skin
Eyes	Stress
Fibromyalgia	Stroke
Fingernails/Hair	Varicose Veins
Headache	

Goldenseal

The United States Department of Veteran Affairs has reported that goldenseal, which normally fights upper respiratory infections, may also be effective in cholesterol lowering. In animal and cell-culture tests at the VA Palo Alto Health Care System senior investigator Jingwen Liu, PhD, found that compounds in goldenseal could lower lipids, thus lowering cholesterol and triglyceride levels. Dr. Liu further stated that unlike statin drugs which can cause liver and muscle damage, goldenseal could be an alternative method of treatment for high cholesterol.

Allergies	Hepatitis
Anemia	Immune System
Asthma	Inflammation
Bronchitis	Influenza
Cancer	Lungs
Cholesterol	Lupus
Circulation	Multiple Sclerosis
Colds	Nervousness
Diabetes	Obesity
Diarrhea	Pancreas
Digestion	Phlegm
Diverticulitis	Shingles
Eyes	Sinus
Gall Stones	Skin
Heartburn	Teeth/Gums
Hemorrhoids	Ulcers

Gotu Kola

Does gotu kola help with energy levels? Researchers at Brigham Young University at Provo, Utah recently did a lab study on herbs that could be beneficial to reduce fatigue and stress. In the study animals were surgically fed gotu kola and cayenne pepper. Fatigue and stress situations were set up. One test for the animals involved swimming in a bucket of cold water, and another was jumping a barrier in order to avoid a mild shock. Within 24 hours the animals fed a combination of gotu kola and cayenne could successfully clear the barrier after being dried off from the cold water. Without the herbs animals took 72 hours to recuperate before clearing the barrier.

Aging
Alzheimer's Disease
Blood Pressure (high)
Energy
Fingernails/Hair
Gall Stones
Heart Disease

Menopause
Obesity
Premenstrual Syndrome
Stroke
Varicose Veins

Hawthorn

In Germany, one of the most prescribed treatments for heart conditions is hawthorn. The University of Maryland Medical Center cites a study of 952 patients with heart failure. The study compared different ways of treating heart failure – with different medications, with hawthorn in combination with drugs and with hawthorn alone. After 2 years, the clinical symptoms decreased significantly in the patients who took hawthorn alone.

Anemia

Arthritis/Joint Pain

Atherosclerosis

Blood Pressure (high)

Cholesterol

Circulation

Diarrhea

Energy

Heart Disease

Immune System

Obesity

Parkinson's Disease

Premenstrual Syndrome

Stroke

Teeth/Gums

Varicose Veins

Hops

Hops has been shown to help menopausal symptoms. Memorial Sloan-Kettering Cancer Center reported a double-blind study from Ghent University in Ghent, Belgium where 67 women, who suffered from menopausal problems, were given either a placebo or hops extract. After the 12 week study the patients who had been given the hops extract showed significant reduction of menopausal discomfort, especially hot flashes.

Anemia

Blood Pressure

Digestion

Headache

Insomnia

Liver

Menopause

Nausea

Nervousness

Obesity

Rheumatism

Stress

Teeth/Gums

Ulcers

"It [the pharmaceutical industry] is the most profitable industry in the world, and partially funds the US government. It surpasses oil in terms of profits and my country recently went to war due to oil pricing. What does that say they will do to keep this other industry in tact? It is up to patients and their families to question what they are being given, and to consumers to demand better, more natural alternatives."

—Margot Kidder, Actress who cured herself
of bipolar with Orthomolecular Medicine.

Horsetail

Horsetail traces its medicinal history back to the ancient Greeks and Romans. One of the more important uses is in its ability to strengthen bones. The Italian medical journal, 'Minerva Ortopedica e Traunatologica', quoted a blind study in which 122 women took part. One third was given a placebo, one third was given Osteosil (a calcium pill) and the final third was given horsetail. After 80 days, the conclusions were that the placebo group showed no change, but the calcium group and the horsetail group showed marked improvement with an average recovery of bone mass of 2.3%.

Aging

Allergies

Arthritis/Joint Pain

Asthma

Atherosclerosis

Bronchitis

Circulation

Cramps

Diabetes

Digestion

Eyes

Fingernails/Hair

Gallbladder

Heart Disease

Inflammation

Kidneys

Lungs

Muscles/Ligaments

Obesity

Osteoporosis

Pancreas

Prostate

Phlegm

Rheumatism

Sinus

Skin

Teeth/Gums

Ulcers

Urinary Tract

Kelp

A new study led by researchers at the University of California in Berkley, California has found that kelp seaweed can be a strong player in the field of cancer-fighting foods. In a lab study, kelp lowered levels of hormones in animals - raising the hope that it would decrease the risk of estrogen-dependent diseases such as breast cancer in humans.

Aging	Kidneys
Anemia	Lungs
Arthritis/Joint Pain	Menopause
Atherosclerosis	Multiple Sclerosis
Breast Cancer	Nausea
Bursitis	Obesity
Cancer	Osteoporosis
Cramps	Premenstrual Syndrome
Depression	Prostate
Diabetes	Radiation exposure
Eyes	Rosacea / Skin
Hypoglycemia	Thyroid/Goiter
Immune System	
Influenza	

Licorice

DGL (deglycyrrhizinated licorice) is a form of licorice from which the compound glycyrrhizin has been removed. The therapeutic effect of DGL has been especially beneficial in the treatment of ulcers, according to Dr. Michael Murray. He cited a study of 40 patients all with chronic duodenal ulcers over a 4 to 12 year period. All of the patients had been referred for surgery because of relentless pain sometimes with frequent vomiting. Half of the patients received 3g of DGL daily for 8 weeks and the other half received 4.5g daily for 16 weeks. All 40 patients showed substantial improvement – usually within 5-7 days and none required surgery during the one year follow-up. Although both doses were effective, the group who received the higher dose showed significant improvement over those who received the lower dose.

Aging

Alzheimer's Disease

Arthritis/Joint Pain

Asthma

Bronchitis

Colds

Constipation

Depression

Digestion

Diverticulitis

Emphysema

Energy

Immune System

Inflammation

Liver

Lungs

Menopause

Pancreas

Phlegm

Pneumonia

Premenstrual Syndrome

Rosacea

Shingles

Teeth/Gums

Ulcers

Milk Thistle

Milk thistle is good for your liver. In 1981 a study done in Finland found that patients with alcoholic liver disease improved liver tissue and reduced liver enzymes after taking milk thistle after only one month. This herb has long been approved by the German Commission E for digestive problems, liver damage and inflammatory liver disease, but a 2006 study revealed that it is also an effective treatment in diabetes. The controlled study, reported in 'Phytotherapy Research', found that milk thistle also lowers blood-glucose levels in type-2 diabetes.

Acne
Aging
Breast Cancer
Cancer
Constipation
Diabetes
Hepatitis
Hypoglycemia
Immune System
Irritable Bowel Syndrome
Liver
Lupus
Menopause
Multiple Sclerosis
Nervousness
Pancreas
Parkinson's Disease
Premenstrual Syndrome
Prostate
Radiation exposure
Rosacea
Shingles
Stress
Ulcerative Colitis
Urinary Tract

Passion Flower

Passionflower has long been known to relieve anxiety and stress and recent studies back up this claim. In 1995, the German Commission E approved passionflower as a treatment for nervous unrest and stated that it was effective in the treatment of anxiety and insomnia. In 2008, the U.S. National Library of Medicine reported a double-blind study on the stress relieving effects of passionflower. Patients at the Dr. Ali Sharati Hospital in Tehran, Iran were given either passionflower or a placebo 90 minutes before surgery. Those who were given the passionflower reported significantly lower anxiety.

Blood Pressure

Headache

Heart Disease

Insomnia

Menopause

Nervousness

Parkinson's Disease

Premenstrual Syndrome

Shingles

Stress

Ulcers

Peppermint

Do you have problems with irritable bowel syndrome? A cup of peppermint tea may help. A research study at the McMaster University in Canada was peer-reviewed in the British Medical Journal on the effects of peppermint and irritable bowel syndrome. The double-blind study included 392 people with IBS who were given either a placebo or peppermint oil. The results were a 57% reduction of symptoms in the patients who were given the peppermint oil.

Alzheimer's Disease
Breast Cancer
Bronchitis
Circulation
Colds
Cramps
Depression
Diarrhea
Digestion
Emphysema
Gallbladder
Gas
Gout
Headache
Heart Disease

Heartburn
Hepatitis
Inflammation
Influenza
Insomnia
Irritable Bowel Syndrome
Liver
Muscles/Ligaments
Nausea
Nervousness
Pain
Phlegm
Premenstrual Syndrome
Shingles
Teeth/Gums

Red Clover

Red clover is another weapon in the fight against cancer. Researchers at Monash University in Victoria, Australia found that an active supplement found in red clover helps prevent prostate cells from advancing to cancerous stages. The results of the study, published in Cancer Epidemiology, Biomarkers and Prevention in December, 2002, found that red clover was five times more effective in fighting cancer cells and early cancer cells.

Acne	Kidneys
Aging	Lungs
Arthritis/Joint Pain	Lupus
Breast Cancer	Multiple Sclerosis
Bronchitis	Nervousness
Cancer	Obesity
Circulation	Pancreas
Colds	Parkinson's Disease
Constipation	Phlegm
Diarrhea	Prostate
Digestion	Prostate Cancer
Diverticulitis	Rheumatism
Gout	Radiation exposure
Hepatitis	Rosacea
Immune System	Shingles
Inflammation	Sinus
Influenza	Skin
Insomnia	Ulcerative Colitis

Red Yeast Rice

According to cardiologist David Becker, a study published in the journal 'Mayo Clinic Proceeding', red yeast rice can help reduce bad cholesterol as effectively as the statin drug Zocor. "This might be an alternative for some people," says cardiologist David Becker, lead author of the study. Becker says he'd been hearing anecdotes for years that red yeast rice was effective in lowering cholesterol — in fact the original statin drugs were derived from a similar yeast. To test this, he put about 35 patients on Zocor (simvastatin). They took 40 milligrams per day. The other 35 volunteers in the study took red yeast rice supplements.

"After 12 weeks, the results were virtually indistinguishable," Becker says. Patients in both groups significantly reduced their cholesterol levels — especially the bad type of cholesterol, called low-density lipoproteins. Becker says the LDL levels for both groups fell by about 40 percent.

Cholesterol

Circulation

Diabetes

Diarrhea

Digestion

Heart Disease

Rosemary

Studies have recently shown that rosemary contains antioxidants that inhibit the action of free radicals – the unstable molecules that are believed to cause many diseases, including cancer. Jim Duke, Ph.D., author of The Green Pharmacy (Rodale, 1997), states the antioxidants in rosemary help to prevent and suppress Alzheimer's disease. "Alzheimer's has been blamed on oxidative and inflammatory processes and on the breakdown or deficiency of choline and acetylcholine in the brain," Duke says. "Rosemary contains more than a dozen antioxidants and a half-dozen compounds reported to prevent the breakdown of acetylcholine." Further Duke says that rosemary is at least as effective as the Alzheimer's drugs currently being administrated and is much easier on the body.

Alzheimer's Disease
Arthritis/Joint Pain
Blood Pressure (high)
Cancer
Cholesterol
Circulation
Colds
Fingernails/Hair
Hair Growth
Headache

Heart Disease
Immune System
Inflammation
Liver
Lungs
Phlegm
Premenstrual Syndrome
Radiation exposure
Rosacea
Shingles

*"Nature is the true healer. The physician
is only nature's assistant."*

— Hippocrates

Sage

Can sage prevent Alzheimer's disease? Researchers at Tehran University Medical Center believes that it's possible. They did a double-blind study of 42 patients with mild to moderate cases of Alzheimer's disease. Each received a daily dose of sage leaf extract or a placebo for four months. The results published in the 'Journal of Clinical Pharmacy and Therapeutics' stated that the patients who received the sage showed significantly better cognitive performance and lower agitation levels than the placebo group.

Acne

Alzheimer's Disease

Anxiety

Breast Pain

Bronchitis

Cancer

Circulation

Colds

Depression

Diabetes

Digestion

Fingernails/Hair

Gas

Headache

Heart Disease

Menopause

Muscles/Ligaments

Nervousness

Phlegm

Rosacea

Shingles

Teeth/Gums

Ulcers

Slippery Elm

Slippery elm gets its name from the mucilage that turns into a gel when it comes into contact with water - coating the throat and the intestinal tract, which can reduce acidity. This is especially helpful for sore throats, coughs, heartburn, colon problems and gastroesophageal reflux disease (GERD) says the University of Michigan Health System. Sloan-Kettering Cancer Center agrees and adds that slippery elm could help to treat diarrhea, indigestion, inflammatory bowel disease and irritable bowel syndrome.

Asthma	Heartburn
Bronchitis	Hemorrhoids
Cancer	Inflammation
Colon	Influenza
Colon Cancer	Irritable Bowel Syndrome
Constipation	Lungs
Cramps	Phlegm
Diarrhea	Pneumonia
Digestion	Ulcerative Colitis
Diverticulitis	Ulcers
Emphysema	
Eyes	

St. John's Wort

Does St. John's Wort really help depression? Several studies have confirmed this. A most recent study was reported in October, 2008 in the 'British Medical Journal'. Klaus Linde at the Centre for Complimentary Medicine in Munich, Germany analyzed twenty-three randomized trials involving 1757 patients suffering from mild to moderate depression. The results showed those patients who took St. John's Wort had a 55% improvement in their symptoms verses those who took a placebo who reported a twenty-two percent improvement.

Anemia

Depression

Diarrhea

Fibromyalgia

Gout

Lungs

Menopause

Nervousness

Shingles

Skin

Ulcers

Urinary Tract

"My opinion, however, is that they (herbs) are superior 95% of the time to any pharmaceutical drug!"

— Dr. Robert E. Willner, M.D.

Tarragon

Tarragon is not only a flavorful culinary spice, but it also helps in the fight against cancer. According to James Duke, Ph.D., a botanist retired from the U.S. Department of Agriculture and author of the 'CRC Handbook of Medicinal Herbs', tarragon contains 72 potential cancer preventatives. In fact, in the comprehensive global analysis of 3100 different foods published in the January 2010 edition of the Nutrition Journal, tarragon was found to have one of the highest antioxidant contents of all the foods studied.

Anemia

Arthritis/Joint Pain

Cancer

Constipation

Cramps

Digestion

Energy

Gas

Insomnia

Liver

Menopause

Nervousness

Skin

Teeth/Gums

Turmeric

Dr. Andrew Weil recently stated that turmeric has been found to be beneficial to help or prevent disease. He cites articles published in the October, 2007 issue of 'Alternative and Complementary Therapies' and summarized in the July 2008 issue of the American Botanical Council publication 'HerbClip' by ethnobotonist James Duke, Ph.D. According to studies, Dr. Duke states turmeric has anti-inflammatory compounds that fight Alzheimer's disease, arthritis and several types of cancer including colon, breast, prostate, liver, esophageal and oral cancer.

Aging	Gas
Allergies	Gout
Alzheimer's Disease	Heart Disease
Arthritis/Joint Pain	Hepatitis
Atherosclerosis	Immune System
Breast Cancer	Inflammation
Bronchitis	Liver
Cancer	Lungs
Cholesterol	Multiple Sclerosis
Circulation	Muscles/Ligaments
Colon Cancer	Nausea
Digestion	Obesity
Fibromyalgia	Pain
Fingernails/Hair	Parkinson's Disease
Gall Stones	Phlegm
Gallbladder	Pneumonia

Prostate

Prostate Cancer

Radiation Exposure

Rheumatism

Rosacea

Sinus

Thyroid /Goiter

Ulcerative Colitis

Ulcers

Uva Ursi

Clinical studies have proven that uva ursi has a positive effect on urinary tract problems. A double-blind study on uva ursi examined the herb's effect on recurrent cystitis in women. Fifty-seven women were divided into two groups – one group taking a placebo and the other group taking a standardized extract of uva ursi. At the end of one year, five of the women in the placebo group had a recurrence of cystitis while none of the uva ursi group had a recurrence. Further, no side effects were reported in either group. Uva ursi is recommended by the German Commission E for use in inflammatory disorders of the urinary tract.

Bronchitis	Menopause
Diabetes	Obesity
Digestion	Pancreas
Hemorrhoids	Phlegm
Hypoglycemia	Prostate
Kidneys	Prostate Cancer
Liver	Urinary Tract

Valerian

A good night's rest is vital for overall health. Unfortunately some people either can't fall asleep or they wake up in the middle of the night. Valerian could solve the problem. A German double-blind study evaluated 121 people with sleep problems for a period of 28 days. Half took a placebo and the other half took 600mg of valerian one hour before bedtime. For the first two weeks there was no significant difference in the groups, but by day twenty-eight, valerian pulled far ahead. 66% percent of the valerian group experienced better sleep compared to 29% of the placebo group.

Acne

Blood Pressure

Colds

Digestion

Emphysema

Fibromyalgia

Gas

Headache

Heart Disease

Heartburn

Hypoglycemia

Insomnia

Menopause

Nervousness

Pain

Premenstrual Syndrome

Stress

Ulcers

Yucca

Problems with stiff joints or inflammation? Yucca could help. A study reported in the 'Journal of Applied Nutrition' (1975 Vol. 27, No.2 and No. 3) reported that Dr. Robert Bingham, the director of the Desert Hot Springs Medical Clinic in Palm Springs, evaluated the use of yucca on 149 arthritic patients. This double-blind study concluded that 60% of the people taking yucca experienced diminished pain, swelling and stiffness compared to the patients receiving the placebo. He told reporters, "'We have known for several years that a food supplement extracted from yucca acts like a natural form of cortisone, to reduce and eliminate the pain, swelling and joint stiffness suffered by arthritis victims. Strong evidence supports the theory that some forms of arthritis may be caused or worsened by toxic substances occurring in the intestines and absorbed by the body. Yucca seems to inhibit these harmful intestinal bacteria and at the same time help the natural and normal forms of bacteria found in the tract."

Arthritis/Joint Pain	Pain
Bursitis	Rheumatism
Gout	Skin
Inflammation	Ulcers

Part III

Health Problems

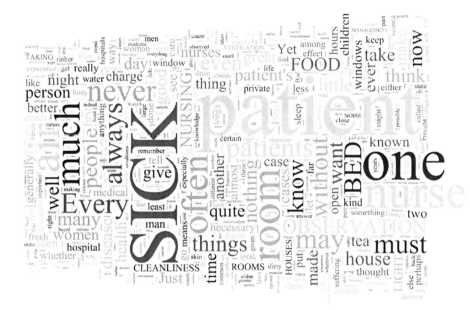

Acne

Healing Foods:

Apple Cider Vinegar	Grapefruit
Apples	Kale
Beans	Kiwi
Brazil Nuts	Lemons/Limes
Broccoli	Lentils
Brown Rice	Oats
Brussels Sprouts	Onions
Cabbage	Oranges
Cantaloupe	Pumpkin/Pumpkin Seeds
Carrots	Spinach
Cherries	Squash
Coconut	Strawberries
Fish	Tomatoes
Flax/flaxseeds	Turnips

Foods to Avoid:

Caffeine	Meat (especially liver)
Chocolate	Nuts
Fried Foods	Shellfish
High-fat Dairy	Sugar

Helpful Herbs & Spices:

Alfalfa	Cayenne Pepper
Aloe Vera	Cloves

Dandelion   Red Clover
Echinacea   Sage
Garlic   Valerian
Milk Thistle

Vitamins & Minerals:

A, B, C, E, F, Niacin, Potassium, Zinc

"Vitality and beauty are gifts of Nature for those who live according to its laws."

— Leonardo DaVinci

Aging

Healing Foods:

Almonds
Apple Cider Vinegar
Apricots
Asparagus
Avocados
Beans
Blueberries
Broccoli
Brown Rice
Brussels Sprouts
Buckwheat Germ
Cabbage
Cauliflower
Cherries
Coconut
Collards
Fish
Flax/Flaxseeds
Grapes

Kale
Lemons & Limes
Lentils
Oats
Olive Oil
Onions
Peppers (Sweet)
Pomegranate
Prunes
Raspberries
Spinach
Strawberries
Swiss Chard
Tomatoes
Turnip (greens)
Walnuts
Watercress
Yogurt

Foods To Avoid:

Artificial Sweeteners
Caffeine
Chocolate

Fried Foods
High-fat Dairy
Potatoes

Preserved Meats   Sugar
Processed Foods   White Flour
Salt   White Rice

Helpful Herbs & Spices:

Aloe Vera   Ginkgo Biloba
Basil   Gotu Kola
Bee Pollen   Horsetail
Cloves   Kelp
Dandelion   Licorice
Echinacea   Milk Thistle
Garlic   Red Clover
Ginger   Turmeric

Vitamins & Minerals:

A, B, C, E, Calcium, Selenium, Zinc

Allergies

Healing Foods:

Apple Cider Vinegar
Apples
Artichokes
Bananas
Beans
Blackberries
Blueberries
Broccoli
Brown Rice
Brussels Sprouts
Cabbage
Carrots
Cauliflower
Cranberries
Fish
Flax/Flaxseeds
Grapefruit

Grapes
Green Tea
Honey
Kale
Lemons/Limes
Onions
Oranges
Peaches
Peas
Peppers (Sweet)
Potatoes
Raspberries
Spinach
Strawberries
Sunflower Seeds
Tomatoes
Yogurt

Foods To Avoid:

Corn
High-fat Dairy
Meat
Nuts

Oats
Soy
Wheat Germ
White Rice

Helpful Herbs & Spices:

Alfalfa   Ginger
Bee Pollen   Ginkgo Biloba
Cardamom   Goldenseal
Chili Pepper   Turmeric
Dandelion
Garlic

Vitamins & Minerals:

A, B3, B12, C, D, E, Calcium, Magnesium, Manganese, Zinc

"If people let government decide what foods they eat and what medicines they take, their bodies will soon be in as sorry a state as are the souls of those who live under tyranny."

Thomas Jefferson

Alzheimer's Disease

Healing Foods:

Almonds

Apples

Apricots

Artichokes

Asparagus

Avocados

Beets

Blackberries

Blackcurrants

Blueberries

Broccoli

Brussels Sprouts

Cabbage

Cantaloupe

Carrots

Cherries

Collards

Cranberries

Dates

Eggs (consume only in moderation)

Fish

Flax/Flaxseeds

Grapefruit

Grapes

Kale

Lemons/Limes

Mango

Oats

Olive Oil

Onions

Oranges

Papaya

Peppers (Sweet)

Pomegranate

Potatoes (with skin)

Prunes

Pumpkin/Pumpkin Seeds

Raspberries

Spinach

Squash

Strawberries

Sweet Potatoes

Swiss Chard

Tomatoes

Walnuts

Watercress

Wheat Germ

Yogurt (Low-fat)

Foods To Avoid:

Aluminum (some baking powders and pancake mixes contain aluminum)

High-fat Dairy

Meat

Processed Meats (especially with nitrates)

Processed Foods

Salt

Sugar

White Flour

White Rice

Helpful Herbs & Spices:

Bee Pollen

Cayenne Pepper

Cinnamon

Dandelion

Garlic

Ginkgo Biloba

Peppermint

Rosemary

Sage

Turmeric

Vitamins & Minerals:

A, B12, C, E, Folate, Niacin, Zinc

Anemia

Healing Foods:

Almonds

Apples

Apricots

Asparagus

Bananas

Beets

Broccoli

Brown Rice

Brussels Sprouts

Carrots

Celery

Dates

Eggs

Figs

Fish

Grapes

Honey

Kale

Lemons/Limes

Lentils

Okra

Oranges

Peas

Prunes

Pumpkin/Pumpkin Seeds

Raisins

Sesame Seeds

Spinach

Squash

Sunflower Seeds

Sweet Potatoes

Swiss Chard

Tomatoes

Turnips (greens)

Walnuts

Watermelon

Foods To Avoid:

Caffeine

Carbonated Beverages

Chocolate

High-fat Dairy

Processed Foods

Soy

Sugar

Helpful Herbs & Spices:

Alfalfa   Kelp
Dandelion   St. Johns Wort
Golden Seal   Tarragon
Hawthorn

Vitamins & Minerals:

B2, B6, B12, Calcium, Copper, Folic Acid, Iron, Manganese, Potassium, Zinc

Arthritis/Joint Pain

Healing Foods:

Almonds

Apple Cider Vinegar

Apples

Artichokes

Asparagus

Avocados

Bananas

Brazil Nuts

Broccoli

Brown Rice

Brussels Sprouts

Cabbage

Cantaloupe

Cauliflower

Celery

Cherries

Collards

Cucumbers

Fish

Flax/Flaxseeds

Grapefruit

Green Tea

Kiwi

Lentils

Lemons

Mango

Mushrooms

Olive Oil

Onions

Oranges

Papaya

Peaches

Pineapple

Pumpkin Seeds

Raisins

Raspberries

Spinach

Squash

Strawberries

Sunflower Seeds

Sweet Potatoes

Walnuts

Foods To Avoid:

Alcohol	Meat (especially red meat)
Caffeine	Peppers (Sweet)
Chocolate	Potatoes
Corn	Processed Foods
Eggplant	Sugar
Fried Foods	Tomatoes
High-fat Dairy	White or Wheat Flour (especially enriched)

Helpful Herbs & Spices:

Alfalfa	Horsetail
Basil	Licorice
Cayenne Pepper	Red Clover
Chili Pepper	Rosemary
Cinnamon	Tarragon
Garlic	Turmeric
Ginger	Yucca

Vitamins & Minerals:

A, B, C, E, F, P, Calcium, Chromium, Magnesium, Niacin, Zinc

"It seems that some consideration should be given to the cause of our mounting physical disabilities, but instead of going to the root of our troubles — wrong habits of eating and drinking — we rush to the medicine shelf and smother our uncomfortable and distressing symptoms under an avalanche of pills, potions and palliatives."

— Brother Roloff

Asthma

Healing Foods:

Apple Cider Vinegar

Beets

Blackberries

Blueberries

Broccoli

Brussels Sprouts

Buckwheat Germ

Cabbage

Cantaloupe

Carrots

Coconut

Collards

Fish

Flax/Flaxseeds

Grapefruit

Green Tea

Honey

Kale

Kiwi

Onions

Oranges

Papaya

Peppers (Sweet)

Raspberries

Spinach

Squash

Strawberries

Swiss Chard

Turnips

Walnuts

Yogurt

Foods To Avoid:

Caffeine

Chocolate

Corn

Eggplant

Eggs

High-fat Dairy

Salt

Soy

Sugar

Sulfites

Tomatoes

Helpful Herbs & Spices:

Basil

Bee Pollen

Cardamom

Cayenne Pepper

Chamomile

Chili Pepper

Echinacea

Garlic

Ginkgo Biloba

Goldenseal

Slippery Elm

Vitamins & Minerals:

A, B3, B6, B12, C, D, E, F, Magnesium, Pantothenic Acid

Atherosclerosis

Healing Foods:

Almonds	Lentils
Asparagus	Mango
Bananas	Oats
Beans	Onions
Blueberries	Oranges
Broccoli	Papaya
Brown Rice	Peaches
Brussels Sprouts	Peppers (Sweet)
Carrots	Persimmon
Cherries	Pomegranate
Fish	Potatoes
Flax/Flaxseeds	Spinach
Grapefruit	Squash
Grapes	Strawberries
Kale	Tomatoes
Kiwi	Walnuts
Lemons/Limes	Wheat Germ

Foods To Avoid:

Eggs	Preserved Meats (especially with nitrates)
Fried Foods	
High-fat Dairy	Processed Foods
Meat	Salt
	Sugar

Helpful Herbs & Spices:

Basil   Hawthorn
Cayenne Pepper   Horsetail
Dandelion   Kelp
Garlic   Turmeric
Ginger

Vitamins & Minerals:

A, B6, B12, C, E, F, P, Calcium, Chromium, CoQ10, Copper, Folic Acid, Inositol, Magnesium, Niacin, Pantothenic Acid, Potassium, Selenium, Zinc

Blood Pressure

Healing Foods:

Almonds
Apple Cider Vinegar
Apples
Apricots
Artichokes
Asparagus
Avocados
Bananas
Beans
Beets
Blackcurrants
Blueberries
Broccoli
Buckwheat Germ
Cabbage
Cantaloupe
Carrots
Cauliflower
Celery
Cranberries
Cucumbers
Eggplant
Figs
Fish

Flax/Flaxseeds
Grapefruit
Grapes
Honey
Kiwi
Lemons/Limes
Lentils
Mango
Mushrooms
Oats
Olive Oil
Onions
Oranges
Peas
Peppers (Sweet)
Pineapple
Potatoes
Prunes
Raisins
Spinach
Squash
Strawberries
Sunflower Seeds
Sweet Potatoes

Tomatoes

Turnips (especially turnip greens)

Walnuts

Watercress

Watermelon

Wheat Germ

Yogurt

Foods To Avoid:

Caffeine

High-fat Dairy

Processed Foods

Processed Meat

Salt

Sugar

Helpful Herbs & Spices (High Blood Pressure):

Cardamom

Cayenne Pepper

Chili Pepper

Dandelion

Garlic

Hawthorn

Hops

Passion Flower

Rosemary

Valerian

(Low Blood Pressure):

Dandelion

Vitamins & Minerals:

A, B3, B6, C, E, K, P, Calcium, Magnesium, Potassium

"Health is a state of complete harmony of the body, mind and spirit. When one is free from physical disabilities and mental distractions, the gates of the soul open."

— B.K.S Iyengar

Bronchitis

Healing Foods:

Apples

Asparagus

Beet (greens)

Blueberries

Broccoli

Cabbage

Cantaloupe

Carrots

Celery

Coconut

Fish

Flax/Flaxseeds

Grapes

Honey

Kale

Mushrooms

Olive Oil

Onions

Oranges

Papaya

Pears

Peppers (Sweet)

Pineapple

Pumpkin/Pumpkin Seeds

Raspberries

Spinach

Squash

Strawberries

Sweet Potatoes

Swiss Chard

Tomatoes

Turnip (greens)

Walnuts

Yogurt

Foods To Avoid:

Caffeine

Corn

Fried Foods

High-fat Dairy

Processed Foods

Salt

Soy

Sugar

Wheat

Helpful Herbs & Spices:

Basil

Cardamom

Cayenne Pepper

Dandelion

Echinacea

Garlic

Ginger

Ginkgo Biloba

Goldenseal

Horsetail

Licorice

Peppermint

Red Clover

Sage

Slippery Elm

Turmeric

Uva Ursi

Vitamins & Minerals:

A, B12, C, E, Zinc

Bursitis

Healing Foods:

Almonds	Grapefruit
Artichokes	Kiwi
Avocados	Oats
Beans	Onions
Broccoli	Oranges
Brown Rice	Papaya
Brussels Sprouts	Peas
Cantaloupe	Pineapple
Carrots	Pumpkin/Pumpkin Seeds
Celery	Strawberries
Collards	Swiss Chard
Fish	Turnips (greens)
Flax Seeds	

Foods To Avoid:

Carbonated Beverages	Processed Foods
Chocolate	Salt
Fried Foods	Sugar
Meat (especially red meat)	Tomatoes

Helpful Herbs & Spices:

Alfalfa	Kelp

Vitamins & Minerals:

A, B, B5, C, D, E, Calcium, Glucosamine, Magnesium,
Selenium

Cancer (General)

Healing Foods:

Almonds	Fish
Apple Cider Vinegar	Flax/Flaxseeds
Apricots	Grapefruit
Asparagus	Grapes
Bananas	Green Tea
Beans	Kale
Beets	Lemons/Limes
Blackcurrants	Lentils
Blueberries	Mango
Brazil Nuts	Mushrooms
Broccoli	Oats
Brown Rice	Okra
Brussels Sprouts	Olive Oil
Buckwheat Germ	Onions
Cabbage	Oranges
Cantaloupe	Papaya
Carrots	Peaches
Cauliflower	Pomegranate
Celery	Pumpkin/Pumpkin Seeds
Cherries	Raisins
Coconut	Rice
Collards	Spinach
Dates	Squash
Eggplant	Strawberries

Sweet Potatoes

Tomatoes

Walnuts

Watercress

Watermelon

Wheat Germ

Yogurt

Foods To Avoid:

Artificial Sweeteners

Charred Foods

Farmed Fish

Food Additives

Fried Foods

High-fat Dairy

Meat (especially smoked meats with nitrates)

Processed Foods

Salt

Sugar

Helpful Herbs & Spices

Bee Pollen

Chili Pepper

Cloves

Dandelion

Echinacea

Garlic

Ginger

Goldenseal

Kelp

Milk Thistle

Red Clover

Rosemary

Sage

Slippery Elm

Tarragon

Turmeric

Vitamins & Minerals:

A, B, C, E, CoQ10, Folate, Iodine, Kelp, Magnesium, Selenium, Zinc

Food and Herbs especially helpful for Radiation Exposure:

Apples

Dandelion

Ginger

Gingko Biloba

Green Tea

Kelp

Milk Thistle

Red Clover

Rosemary

Sunflower Seeds

Tumeric

Foods /Herbs/Spices especially helpful for the following types of Cancer:

Breast Cancer:

Apples	Lemons/Limes
Broccoli	Mango
Brussels Sprouts	Milk Thistle
Cabbage	Olive Oil
Carrots	Onions
Cauliflower	Papaya
Cloves	Peaches
Coconut	Peppermint
Corn	Pomegranate
Dandelion	Red Clover
Echinacea	Spinach
Flax/Flaxseeds	Strawberries
Garlic	Sweet Potatoes
Ginger	Tomatoes
Ginkgo Biloba	Turmeric
Green Tea	Watercress
Kale	Wheat Germ
Kelp	

Cervical Cancer:

Apples	Broccoli
Asparagus	Cabbage

Carrots   Pumpkin
Onions   Spinach
Papaya   Tomatoes

Colon Cancer:

Asparagus   Green Tea
Bananas   Kale
Beans   Lemons/Limes
Beets   Lentils
Broccoli   Mango
Brussels Sprouts   Oats
Buckwheat Germ   Okra
Cabbage   Onions
Carrots   Oranges
Cauliflower   Papaya
Celery   Spinach
Coconut   Squash
Figs   Strawberries
Fish   Sweet Potatoes
Flaxseeds   Turmeric
Garlic   Walnuts
Grapefruit   Wheat Germ
Grapes

Esophageal Cancer:

Broccoli   Carrots
Brussels Sprouts   Cauliflower
Cabbage   Green Tea

Kale   Swiss Chard
Oats   Wheat Germ

Lung Cancer:

Asparagus   Collards
Beans   Lemons/Limes
Beets   Lentils
Broccoli   Oranges
Buckwheat Germ   Papaya
Cabbage   Pumpkin
Carrots   Spinach
Cauliflower   Squash

Pancreatic Cancer:

Broccoli   Cauliflower
Brussels Sprouts   Flax/Flaxseeds
Cabbage   Green Tea

Prostate Cancer:

Carrots   Onions
Cauliflower   Papaya
Cloves   Pomegranate
Dandelion   Squash
Echinacea   Tomatoes
Flax/Flaxseeds   Turmeric
Garlic   Uva Ursi
Grapefruit   Walnuts
Green Tea

Skin Cancer:

Aloe Vera

Beets

Brazil Nuts

Chili Peppers

Fish

Green Tea

Lemons/Limes

Pomegranate

Sweet Potatoes

Tomatoes

Walnuts

Stomach Cancer:

Apples

Broccoli

Brown Rice

Celery

Dates

Garlic

Ginger

Grapefruit

Grapes

Green Tea

Lemons/Limes

Oats

Oranges

Sweet Potatoes

Tomatoes

Wheat

Uterine Cancer:

Cabbage

Carrots

Cranberries

Onions

Oranges

Papaya

Peppers, (Sweet)

Raspberries

Squash

Strawberries

Tomatoes

Yogurt

"The work of the doctor will, in the future, be ever more that of an educator, and ever less that of a man who treats ailments."

— Lord Horder

Cholesterol

Healing Foods:

Almonds

Apple Cider Vinegar

Apples

Artichokes

Asparagus

Avocados

Bananas

Beans

Beets

Cantaloupe

Cherries

Corn

Eggplant

Fish

Flax/Flaxseeds

Garlic

Grapefruit

Green Tea

Lemons/Limes

Lentils

Mushrooms

Oats

Olive Oil

Onions

Pears

Peas

Persimmons

Pomegranate

Prunes

Pumpkin/Pumpkin Seeds

Raisins

Sesame Seeds

Sunflower Seeds

Tomatoes

Walnuts

Watercress

Watermelon

Wheat Germ

Yogurt

Foods To Avoid:

Eggs   Meat
Fried Foods   Processed Meat
High Fat Dairy   Sugar

Helpful Herbs & Spices:

Alfalfa   Ginger
Basil   Goldenseal
Chili Pepper   Red Yeast Rice
Cinnamon   Rosemary
Cloves   Turmeric
Garlic

Vitamins & Minerals:

A, B3, B6, B12, C, D, E, Biotin, Calcium, CoQ10, Folic Acid, Iodine, Iron, Lecithin, Magnesium, Potassium

Circulation

Healing Foods:

Almonds	Lentils
Apples	Onions
Apricots	Oranges
Avocados	Peppers (Sweet)
Beans	Pineapple
Beets	Pomegranate
Blackcurrants	Prunes
Broccoli	Pumpkin/Pumpkin Seeds
Carrots	Spinach
Collards	Strawberries
Eggplant	Sunflower Seeds
Fish	Sweet Potatoes
Flax/Flaxseeds	Tomatoes
Grapefruit	Walnuts
Grapes	Watercress
Green Tea	Watermelon
Kiwi	Wheat Germ
Lemons/Limes	Yogurt

Foods To Avoid:

Carbonated Beverages	Processed Meat
Chocolate	Salt
Meat	Sugar

Helpful Herbs & Spices:

Basil	Goldenseal
Cardamom	Hawthorn
Cayenne Pepper	Horsetail
Chili Pepper	Red Clover
Cinnamon	Red Yeast Rice
Dandelion	Rosemary
Garlic	Sage
Ginger	Turmeric
Ginkgo Biloba	

Vitamins & Minerals:

A, B3, C, D, E, Calcium, Lecithin, Magnesium, Potassium

Colds

Healing Foods:

Apple Cider Vinegar

Apples

Bananas

Blackcurrants

Blueberries

Broccoli

Brown Rice

Brussels Sprouts

Carrots

Cauliflower

Celery

Cherries

Coconut

Collards

Cranberries

Eggplant

Eggs

Fish

Grapefruit

Grapes

Green Tea

Honey

Kale

Kiwi

Lemons/Limes

Mango

Oats

Onions

Oranges

Papaya

Pears

Peas

Peppers (Sweet)

Pineapple

Raspberries

Spinach

Squash

Strawberries

Sweet Potatoes

Tomatoes

Turnips (especially turnip greens)

Watercress

Yogurt

Foods To Avoid:

Caffeine   Meat (especially red meat)
Chocolate   Salt
Dairy   Sugar

Helpful Herbs & Spices:

Basil   Garlic
Cayenne Pepper   Ginger
Chamomile   Goldenseal
Chili Pepper   Red Clover
Cinnamon   Rosemary
Cloves   Sage
Echinacea   Valerian

Vitamins & Minerals:

A, B, B3, C, D, E, F, Calcium, Lysine, Pantothenic Acid

Colon

Healing Foods:

Almonds

Apples

Apricots

Asparagus

Bananas

Beans

Beets

Broccoli

Brown RIce

Brussels Sprouts

Buckwheat Germ

Cabbage

Carrots

Cauliflower

Celery

Coconut

Figs

Fish

Flax/Flaxseeds

Grapefruit

Grapes

Green Tea

Honey

Kale

Lentils

Mango

Oats

Okra

Onions

Oranges

Papaya

Peaches

Pears

Peas

Prunes

Spinach

Squash

Strawberries

Sunflower Seeds

Sweet Potatoes

Tomatoes

Turnips

Walnuts

Wheat

Yogurt

Foods To Avoid:

Caffeine   Processed Foods
Carbonated Beverages   Red Meat
High-fat Dairy   Sugar

Helpful Herbs & Spices:

Alfalfa   Ginger
Aloe Vera   Slippery Elm
Cinnamon   Turmeric
Garlic

Vitamins & Minerals:

A, B6, B12, C, D, E, K, Calcium

Constipation

Healing Foods:

Almonds
Apple Cider Vinegar
Apples
Apricots
Asparagus
Avocados
Bananas
Beans
Beets
Blackberries
Blueberries
Broccoli
Brown Rice
Brussels Sprouts
Buckwheat Germ
Cabbage
Carrots
Cauliflower
Celery
Coconut
Collards
Corn
Cucumber
Figs

Flax/Flaxseeds
Grapes
Kale
Kiwi
Lemons/Limes
Lentils
Mango
Oats
Oranges
Peaches
Pears
Peas
Peppers (Sweet)
Potatoes (with skin)
Prunes
Pumpkin/Pumpkin Seeds
Raisins
Raspberries
Spinach
Squash
Strawberries
Sunflower Seeds
Sweet Potatoes
Swiss Chard

Tomatoes   Wheat Germ
Turnip (greens)   Yogurt

Foods To Avoid:

High-fat Dairy   Processed Food
Meat   Sugar

Helpful Herbs & Spices:

Alfalfa   Milk Thistle
Aloe Vera   Red Clover
Basil   Slippery Elm
Dandelion   Tarragon
Licorice

Vitamins & Minerals:

B12, C, D, E, Calcium, Potassium

Cramps

Healing Foods:

Almonds

Apple Cider Vinegar

Apples

Apricots

Artichokes

Avocados

Bananas

Beans

Broccoli

Brussels Sprouts

Cabbage

Cantaloupe

Cauliflower

Collards

Dates

Figs

Fish

Flax/Flaxseeds

Grapefruit

Kale

Kiwi

Oranges

Pears

Peas

Potatoes

Prunes

Raisins

Spinach

Squash

Strawberries

Sunflower Seeds

Swiss Chard

Tomatoes

Foods To Avoid:

Caffeine

Carbonated Beverages

Chocolate

Dairy Products

Meat

Helpful Herbs & Spices:

Alfalfa   Ginger
Basil   Ginkgo Biloba
Cardamom   Horsetail
Cayenne Pepper   Kelp
Chamomile   Peppermint
Cloves   Slippery Elm
Dandelion   Tarragon
Garlic

Vitamins & Minerals:

B6, C, D, E, Calcium, Magnesium, Potassium

"…Though scientists do not agree till now on the relationship between illness and nutrition, but evidence is mounting and there is a general consensus that the quality and quantity of foods we consume in our affluent society and our sedentary lifestyle are the main factors causing many forms of cancer, cardiovascular and other degenerative diseases…"

—Dr. Ted Cooper, Former US Assistant Health Secretary

Depression

Healing Foods:

Asparagus

Bananas

Beans

Broccoli

Brown Rice

Brussels Sprouts

Cabbage

Cauliflower

Collards

Eggs

Fish

Flax/Flaxseeds

Kale

Kiwi

Lemons/Limes

Low-fat Dairy

Olive Oil

Oranges

Peas

Prunes

Pumpkin/Pumpkin Seeds

Spinach

Strawberries

Sunflower Seeds

Turnips

Walnuts

Wheat Germ

Foods To Avoid:

Alcohol

Artificial Sweeteners

Caffeine

Fried Foods

High-fat Dairy

Processed Foods

Sugar

White Flour

White Rice

Helpful Herbs & Spices:

Basil	Ginkgo Biloba
Chili Pepper	Kelp
Cloves	Peppermint
Garlic	Sage
Ginger	St. Johns Wort

Vitamins & Minerals:

B1, B2, B6, B12, C, E, Calcium, Copper Folate, Iodine, Iron, Magnesium, Potassium

Diabetes

Healing Foods:

Almonds
Apple Cider Vinegar
Artichokes
Asparagus
Avocados
Beans
Blackcurrants
Blueberries
Brazil Nuts
Broccoli
Brown Rice
Buckwheat Germ
Cabbage
Cauliflower
Cherries
Coconut
Collards
Eggplant

Fish
Flax/Flaxseeds
Grapefruit
Kale
Lemons/Limes
Lentils
Oats
Olive Oil
Pomegranate
Pumpkin/Pumpkin Seeds
Raspberries
Spinach
Strawberries
Sweet Potatoes
Swiss Chard
Tomatoes
Walnuts
Wheat Germ

Foods To Avoid:

Bananas (especially ripe)
Beets
Chocolate

Corn
Dates
Eggs

Fried Foods

Grapes

High-fat Dairy

Honey

Mango

Potatoes

Processed Foods

Processed Meat

Raisins

Salt

Squash

Sugar

Turnips

Watermelon

White Flour

Helpful Herbs & Spices:

Alfalfa

Cayenne Pepper

Cinnamon

Cloves

Dandelion

Goldenseal

Horsetail

Kelp

Milk Thistle

Red Yeast Rice

Sage

Uva Ursi

Vitamins & Minerals:

A, B3, B6, B12, C, E, P, Chromium, Choline, Inositol, Potassium

"Leave your drugs in the chemist's pot if you can heal the patient with food."

— Hippocrates

Diarrhea

Healing Foods:

Apple Cider Vinegar	Dates
Apples	Green Tea
Applesauce	Oranges
Bananas	Persimmons
Beets (also beet greens)	Pineapple
Blackberries	Pomegranate
Blackcurrants	Potatoes
Blueberries	Rice
Brown Rice	Squash
Carrots	Yogurt

Foods To Avoid:

Alcohol	Cauliflower
Beans	Dairy Products
Broccoli	Fried Foods
Cabbage	Onions
Carbonated Beverages	Peas

Helpful Herbs & Spices

Cayenne Pepper	Goldenseal
Cinnamon	Hawthorn
Garlic	Peppermint
Ginger	Red Clover

Red Yeast Rice   St. Johns Wort
Slippery Elm

Vitamins & Minerals:

B, B2, Niacin, Potassium

Digestion

Healing Foods:

Artichokes

Bananas

Beets

Brown Rice

Buckwheat Germ

Carrots

Coconut

Collards

Cucumbers

Flax/Flaxseeds

Honey

Mango

Papaya

Peaches

Pears

Pineapple

Raisins

Raspberries

Spinach

Strawberries

Sunflower Seeds

Sweet Potatoes

Turnips

Walnuts

Wheat Germ

Yogurt

Foods To Avoid:

Beans

Broccoli

Brussels Sprouts

Cabbage

Caffeine

Chili Peppers

Chocolate

Dairy Products

Foods Additives
(including artificial sugar)

Fried Food

Grapefruit

High-fat Dairy

Lemons/Limes

Meat (especially red meat)

Onions   Tomatoes

Oranges

Helpful Herbs & Spices:

Alfalfa   Goldenseal

Aloe Vera   Hops

Basil   Horsetail

Bee Pollen   Licorice

Cardamom   Peppermint

Cayenne Pepper   Red Yeast Rice

Chamomile   Sage

Chili Pepper   Slippery Elm

Cinnamon   Tarragon

Cloves   Turmeric

Dandelion   Uva Ursi

Garlic   Valerian

Ginger

Vitamins & Minerals:

A, B1, B3, B12, Biotin, Potassium, Zinc

"And we have made of ourselves living cesspools, and driven doctors to invent names for our diseases."

— Plato

Diverticulitis

Healing Foods:

Apples	Grapes
Apricots	Kale
Artichokes	Lentils
Asparagus	Mushrooms
Bananas	Oats
Beans	Onions
Beets	Oranges
Blueberries	Peaches
Broccoli	Pears
Brown Rice	Peas
Brussels Sprouts	Peppers (Sweet)
Cabbage	Pineapple
Cantaloupe	Potatoes
Carrots	Prunes
Celery	Sweet Potatoes
Cherries	Swiss Chard
Eggplant	Turnips (especially greens)
Fish	Wheat Germ
Grapefruit	Yogurt

Foods To Avoid:

Almonds	Brazil Nuts
Blackberries	Chili Peppers

Cucumber
Dried Fruit
Flax Seeds
Raisins
Raspberries
Sesame Seeds
Sunflower Seeds

Spicy Foods
Squash
Strawberries
Sugar
Tomatoes
Walnuts
Watermelon

Helpful Herbs & Spices:

Alfalfa
Aloe Vera
Chamomile
Cloves
Garlic

Goldenseal
Licorice
Red Clover
Slippery Elm

Vitamins:

B, C, E

Emphysema

Healing Foods:

Apricots	Lemons/Limes
Asparagus	Mango
Avocados	Onions
Beets	Oranges
Blueberries	Papaya
Broccoli	Peaches
Brown Rice	Pears
Brussels Sprouts	Pineapple
Carrots	Potatoes
Celery	Raspberries
Cherries	Spinach
Collards	Squash
Flax/Flaxseeds	Strawberries
Grapefruit	Sweet Potatoes
Grapes	Tomatoes
Green Tea	Watercress
Kale	Wheat Germ
Kiwi	

Foods To Avoid:

Alcohol	Bananas
Apples	Beans
Artificial Sweeteners	Cabbage

Caffeine

Cauliflower

Corn

Cucumbers

Dates

Dried Fruit

Eggs

Figs

Fried Foods

High Fat Dairy

Lentils

Meat (especially red meat)

Peas

Peppers (Sweet)

Persimmons

Processed Foods

Raisins

Salt

Sugar

Turnips

White Flour

Helpful Herbs & Spices:

Aloe Vera

Basil

Chile Pepper

Dandelion

Garlic

Ginger

Licorice

Peppermint

Slippery Elm

Valerian

Vitamins & Minerals:

A, B6, C, E, Biotin, Glutathione, Magnesium, Niacin, Potassium, Zinc

"Health requires healthy food. One of the biggest tragedies of human civilization is the precedents of chemical therapy over nutrition. It's a substitution of artificial therapy over nature, of poisons over food, in which we are feeding people poisons trying to correct the reactions of starvation."

— Dr. Royal Lee

Energy

Healing Foods:

Almonds

Apple Cider Vinegar

Avocados

Bananas

Beans

Beets

Blackberries

Blackcurrants

Blueberries

Brazil Nuts

Broccoli

Brown Rice

Cauliflower

Celery

Coconut

Collards

Corn

Dates

Eggs

Figs

Fish

Flax/Flaxseeds

Grapes

Honey

Kale

Oats

Papaya

Peppers (Sweet)

Raisins

Raspberries

Spinach

Swiss Chard

Walnuts

Wheat Germ

Foods To Avoid:

Alcohol

Artificial Sweeteners

Dairy

Fried Foods

Processed Meat

Sugar

Helpful Herbs & Spices:

Alfalfa   Gotu Kola

Bee Pollen   Hawthorn

Cardamom   Licorice

Cayenne Pepper   Tarragon

Dandelion

Vitamins & Minerals:

A, B6, B12, C, E, D, F, K, Biotin, Choline, Iron, Paba, Potassium, Riboflavin, Thiamine, Zinc

Eyes

Healing Foods:

Almonds

Apple Cider Vinegar

Apples

Apricots

Asparagus

Avocados

Bananas

Beans

Beets

Blackcurrants

Blueberries

Brazil Nuts

Broccoli

Brown Rice

Brussels Sprouts

Cabbage

Cantaloupe

Carrots

Celery

Cherries

Collards

Corn

Cranberries

Cucumbers

Eggs

Fish

Flax/Flaxseeds

Grapefruit

Grapes

Kale

Kiwi

Lemons/Limes

Mango

Oats

Olive Oil

Onions

Oranges

Papaya

Peas

Peppers (Sweet)

Pineapple

Pumpkin/Pumpkin Seeds

Raisins

Raspberries

Spinach

Squash

Strawberries

Sunflower Seeds

Sweet Potatoes   Wheat Germ

Tomatoes   Yogurt

Walnuts

Foods To Avoid:

Fried Foods   Salt

High Fat Dairy   Sugar

Processed Meat

Helpful Herbs & Spices:

Basil   Goldenseal

Cayenne Pepper   Horsetail

Chamomile   Kelp

Garlic   Slippery Elm

Ginkgo Biloba

Vitamins & Minerals:

A, B, C, CoQ10, D, E, Inositol, Selenium, Riboflavin, Zinc

Fibromyalgia

Healing Foods:

Almonds
Apple Cider Vinegar
Apples
Artichokes
Asparagus
Beets
Blueberries
Brazil Nuts
Broccoli
Brussels Sprouts
Carrots
Celery
Collards
Fish
Garlic

Grapes
Kale
Kiwi
Lemons/Limes
Lentils
Onions
Pumpkin/Pumpkin Seeds
Sesame Seeds
Spinach
Squash
Sunflower Seeds
Sweet Potatoes
Swiss Chard
Walnuts
Yogurt

Foods To Avoid:

Artificial Sweeteners
Bananas
Beans
Brown Rice
Caffeine
Carbonated Beverages

Chocolate
Corn
Dried Fruit
Eggplant
Eggs
Food Additives

Fried Foods

Fruit Juices

High-fat Dairy

Mango

Mushrooms

Oats

Oranges

Peppers (Sweet)

Potatoes

Raisins

Strawberries

Sugar

Tomatoes

Watermelon

Wheat Germ

White Flour

Helpful Herbs & Spices:

Cayenne

Chamomile

Dandelion

Echinacea

Garlic

Ginger

Goldenseal

Passionflower

St. John's Wort

Tumeric

Valerian

Vitamins & Minerals:

A, B1, B2, B3, B5, B6, B12, C, CoQ10, E, Calcium, Magnesium, Potassium

Fingernails/Hair

Healing Foods:

Almonds

Apple Cider Vinegar

Asparagus

Beans

Brazil Nuts

Broccoli

Brown Rice

Brussels Sprouts

Carrots

Coconut

Collards

Eggs

Fish

Flax/Flax Seeds

Kale

Lentils

Low-fat Dairy

Onions

Oranges

Papaya

Peppers (Sweet)

Pumpkin/Pumpkin Seeds

Spinach

Squash

Sweet Potatoes

Swiss Chard

Walnuts

Wheat Germ

Yogurt

Foods To Avoid:

Caffeine

Fried Foods

Processed Foods

Salt

Sugar

Helpful Herbs & Spices:

Alfalfa	Horsetail
Dandelion	Rosemary
Ginkgo Biloba	Sage
Gotu Kola	Turmeric

Vitamins & Minerals:

A, B12, C, D, E, Biotin, Calcium, Iodine, Iron, Niacin, Zinc

Gall Stones

Healing Foods:

Almonds	Grapefruit
Apple Cider Vinegar	Kale
Apples	Kiwi
Apricots	Lentils
Artichokes	Oats
Asparagus	Olive Oil
Avocados	Oranges
Blackberries	Pears
Blueberries	Pomegranate
Brazil Nuts	Prunes
Broccoli	Raisins
Brown Rice	Raspberries
Brussels Sprouts	Strawberries
Cantaloupe	Sweet Potatoes
Carrots	Walnuts
Celery	Watermelon
Cherries	Wheat Germ
Flax/Flaxseeds	Yogurt

Foods To Avoid:

Alcohol (especially cocktails and hard liquor)	Cabbage
	Caffeine
Artificial Sweetener	Carbonated Beverages
Beans	

Cauliflower

Meat (especially red meat)

Chocolate

Onions

Corn

Processed Foods

Eggs

Salt

Food Additives

Sugar

Fried Foods

White Flour

High-fat Dairy

Helpful Herbs & Spices:

Dandelion

Goldenseal

Garlic

Gotu Kola

Ginger

Turmeric

Vitamins & Minerals:

B, C, D, E, Inositol, Magnesium

"What most people do not know is that the only thing that drugs do is alleviate the symptoms, and that they do not help in regaining the body's health and well being. Drugs do not cure. Nature and nutrition do."

—Dr. Bernard Jensen

Gallbladder

Healing Foods:

Apple Cider Vinegar

Apples

Apricots

Artichokes

Avocados

Beans

Beets (and beet greens)

Blackberries

Blueberries

Blackcurrants

Cantaloupe

Carrots

Celery

Coconut

Cucumbers

Figs

Fish

Flax Seeds

Garlic

Grapes

Lemons/Limes

Okra

Papaya

Pears

Prunes

Raspberries

Strawberries

Sweet Potatoes

Swiss Chard

Tomatoes

Foods To Avoid:

Cabbage

Caffeine

Carbonated Beverages

Cauliflower

Chili Peppers

Chocolate

Dairy Products

Eggs

Fried Foods

Grapefruit

High-fat Dairy

Meat (especially red meat)

Nuts

Oats

Onions

Oranges

Processed Foods

Spicy Foods

Sugar

Turnips

Wheat Germ

White Flour

Helpful Herbs & Spices:

Alfalfa

Dandelion

Ginger

Horsetail

Parley

Peppermint

Turmeric

Vitamins & Minerals:

A, B1, B3, B6, C, E, F, Calcium

Gas

Healing Foods:

Beets (especially greens)

Carrots

Cherries

Collards

Fish

Flax/Flaxseeds

Grapes

Kale

Kiwi

Pineapple

Pumpkin

Spinach

Swiss Chard

Wheat Germ

Yogurt

Foods To Avoid:

Apples

Apricots

Beans

Broccoli

Brussels Sprouts

Cabbage

Cantaloupe

Carbonated Beverages

Cauliflower

Celery

Corn

Cucumbers

Dairy Products

Eggs

Lentils

Nuts

Oats

Okra

Onions

Oranges

Peaches

Pears

Peas

Peppers (Sweet)

Potatoes

Raisins

Turnips

Helpful Herbs & Spices:

Basil	Peppermint
Cardamom	Sage
Chamomile	Tarragon
Cinnamon	Turmeric
Cloves	Valerian
Ginger	

Vitamins:

A, B12, C, D, E

Gout

Healing Foods:

Almonds

Apple Cider Vinegar

Apples

Bananas

Beets (especially beet greens)

Blackberries

Blueberries

Brown Rice

Buckwheat Germ

Cabbage

Cantaloupe

Carrots

Celery

Cherries

Cranberry

Cucumber

Eggs

Fish

Flax/Flaxseeds

Grapes

Green Tea

Kale

Lemons/Limes

Oranges

Peppers (Sweet)

Pineapple

Potatoes

Pumpkin/Pumpkin Seeds

Strawberries

Tomatoes

Turnips (especially turnip greens)

Yogurt

Foods To Avoid:

Alcohol

Asparagus

Beans

Cauliflower

Lentils

Meat (especially red meat)

Mushrooms

Peas

Spinach

Sugar

White Flour

Helpful Herbs & Spices:

Alfalfa	Red Clover
Dandelion	St. Johns Wort
Ginger	Turmeric
Peppermint	Yucca

Vitamins & Minerals:

B, C, E, Calcium, Magnesium, Potassium, Selenium

"All that man needs for health and healing has been provided by God in nature, the challenge of science is to find it."

—Philippus Theophrastrus Bombast that of Aureolus Paracelsus (1493-1541)

Headache

Healing Foods:

Apple Cider Vinegar

Beans

Broccoli

Brown Rice

Carrots

Celery

Cherries

Collards

Cranberries

Fish

Garlic

Kale

Oats

Pears

Pineapple

Spinach

Squash

Sweet Potatoes

Swiss Chard

Watercress

Foods To Avoid:

Artificial Sweeteners

Avocados

Bananas

Cabbage

Chocolate

Dairy (especially aged cheeses)

Dates

Figs

Fried Foods

Lemons/Limes

Meat (processed or smoked meat)

Nuts

Onions

Oranges

Processed Foods

Raisins

Raspberries

Salt

Seeds (sunflower or sesame)

Sugar   Wheat Germ
Tomatoes

Helpful Herbs & Spices:

Basil   Hops
Cayenne Pepper   Passion Flower
Chamomile   Peppermint
Cinnamon   Rosemary
Garlic   Sage
Ginger   Valerian
Ginkgo Biloba

Vitamins & Minerals:

A, B6, B12, C, Calcium, CoQ10, Magnesium, Potassium

Heart Disease

Healing Foods:

Almonds

Apples

Apricots

Artichokes

Asparagus

Avocados

Bananas

Beans

Beets

Blackcurrants

Blueberries

Brazil Nuts

Broccoli

Brown Rice

Buckwheat Germ

Cabbage

Cantaloupe

Carrots

Cauliflower

Cherries

Coconut

Collards

Dates

Fish

Flax/Flaxseeds

Grapefruit

Grapes

Green Tea

Honey

Kale

Lemons/Limes

Lentils

Oats

Okra

Olive Oil

Onions

Oranges

Papaya

Peppers (Sweet)

Persimmons

Pineapple

Pomegranate

Potatoes

Prunes

Pumpkin/Pumpkin Seeds

Raisins

Sesame Seeds

Spinach

Squash
Strawberries
Sunflower Seeds
Sweet Potatoes
Tomatoes

Walnuts
Watermelon
Wheat Germ
Yogurt

Foods To Avoid:

Fried Foods
High-fat Dairy
Meat (especially red meat)

Processed foods
Salt
Sugar

Helpful Herbs & Spices:

Alfalfa
Basil
Cayenne Pepper
Chili Pepper
Cinnamon
Garlic
Ginger
Ginkgo Biloba
Gotu Kola

Hawthorn
Horsetail
Passion Flower
Peppermint
Red Yeast Rice
Rosemary
Sage
Turmeric
Valerian

Vitamins & Minerals:

A, B, C, D, E, Biotin, Calcium, Inositol, Iodine, Iron, Lecithin, Magnesium, Potassium, Thiamine

"God, in His infinite wisdom, neglected nothing and if we would eat our food without trying to improve, change or refine it, thereby destroying its life-giving elements, it would meet all requirements of the body."

— Jethro Kloss

Heartburn

Healing Foods:

Apple Cider Vinegar	Fish
Apples	Grapes
Asparagus	Honey
Avocados	Low-fat Dairy
Bananas	Oats
Broccoli	Papaya
Brown Rice	Peas
Cabbage	Pineapple
Carrots	Potatoes
Eggs	Wheat Germ

Foods to Avoid:

Caffeine	Meat
Cranberries	Onions
Fried Foods	Oranges
Grapefruit	Salt
High-fat Dairy	Sugar
Lemons/Limes	Tomatoes

Helpful Herbs & Spices:

Aloe Vera	Cinnamon
Cayenne Pepper	Dandelion

Ginger   Peppermint
Goldenseal   Slippery Elm

Vitamins & Minerals:

A, B3, C, K, Biotin, Calcium, Potassium, Zinc

Hemorrhoids

Healing Foods:

Almonds

Apple Cider Vinegar

Apples (especially juice)

Apricots

Bananas

Beans (especially lima beans)

Beets

Blackberries (especially juice)

Blueberries (especially juice)

Broccoli (cooked)

Brown Rice

Buckwheat Germ

Cabbage

Cantaloupe

Carrots

Cherries (especially juice)

Coconut

Figs

Fish

Flax/Flaxseeds

Kale

Oats

Olive Oil

Onions

Oranges

Papaya

Peaches

Pears

Peas

Pomegranate

Potatoes

Prunes

Pumpkin/Pumpkin Seeds

Raisins

Sesame Seeds

Spinach

Sunflower Seeds

Sweet Potatoes

Swiss Chard (cooked)

Wheat Germ

Foods To Avoid:

Caffeine

Dairy

Eggs

Meat (especially red meat)

Processed Foods   Spicy Foods

Salt   Sugar

Helpful Herbs & Spices:

Aloe Vera   Goldenseal

Cayenne Pepper   Slippery Elm

Chamomile   Uva Ursi

Garlic   White Oak Bark

Ginger

Vitamins & Minerals:

A, B1, B3, B6, C, E, Lecithin, Potassium

Hepatitis

Healing Foods:

Apples
Artichokes
Asparagus
Beans
Beets
Blackberries
Blackcurrants
Blueberries
Brazil Nuts
Broccoli
Brown Rice
Cabbage
Cantaloupe
Carrots
Cauliflower
Celery
Coconut
Fish

Flax/Flaxseeds
Grapes
Kale
Lemons/Limes
Oats
Oranges
Papaya
Potatoes
Radish
Raspberries
Spinach
Squash
Strawberries
Sweet Potatoes
Tomatoes
Walnuts
Wheat Germ
Yogurt

Foods To Avoid:

Alcohol
Caffeine
Chili Peppers

Eggs
Fried Foods
High-fat Dairy

Honey

Meat

Onions

Processed Foods

Salt

Sugar

Helpful Herbs & Spices:

Chamomile

Cloves

Dandelion

Garlic

Ginger

Goldenseal

Milk Thistle

Peppermint

Red Clover

Turmeric

Vitamins & Minerals:

A, B12, C, D, E, Choline, Folic Acid, Niacin, Pantothenic Acid, Thiamine, Riboflavin, Zinc

Hypoglycemia

Healing Foods:

Avocados

Beans

Blackberries

Blueberries

Broccoli

Brown Rice

Brussels Sprouts

Cabbage

Carrots

Cauliflower

Celery

Cherries

Cucumbers

Fish

Kale

Mushrooms

Oats

Onions

Oranges

Pears

Peppers (Sweet)

Spinach

Squash

Strawberries

Swiss Chard

Tomatoes

Yogurt

Foods To Avoid:

Alcohol

Caffeine

Carbonated Beverages

Chocolate

Dried Fruit

Fried Foods

Fruit Juices

High-fat Dairy

Processed Foods

Processed Meats

Sugar

White Flour

Helpful Herbs & Spices:

Bee Pollen   Uva Ursi
Kelp   Valerian
Milk Thistle

Vitamins & Minerals:

B6, B12, Chromium, Magnesium, Manganese, Zinc

"At the end of times the merchants of the word will deceive the nations of the world through Their Pharmacia."

— Revelations 18:23

Immune System

Healing Foods:

Almonds

Asparagus

Beans

Blackberries

Blueberries

Broccoli

Brown Rice

Buckwheat Germ

Cabbage

Cantaloupe

Carrots

Cauliflower

Collards

Fish

Flax/Flaxseeds

Grapefruit

Green Tea

Kale

Kiwi

Mushrooms

Oats

Onions

Oranges

Papaya

Peppers (Sweet)

Pomegranate

Pumpkin/Pumpkin Seeds

Raspberries

Spinach

Squash

Strawberries

Sweet Potatoes

Tomatoes

Turnips (greens)

Walnuts

Yogurt

Foods To Avoid:

Alcohol

Artificial Sweeteners

Caffeine

Carbonated Beverages

Food Additives

Fried Foods

Meat   Processed Meat
Processed Foods   Sugar

Helpful Herbs & Spices:

Bee Pollen   Ginger
Cayenne Pepper   Ginkgo Biloba
Chamomile   Goldenseal
Chili Pepper   Kelp
Cinnamon   Licorice
Cloves   Milk Thistle
Dandelion   Red Clover
Echinacea   Rosemary
Garlic   Turmeric

Vitamins & Minerals:

A, B6, C, D, E, K, Copper, Iron, Manganese, Selenium, Zinc

Inflammation

Healing Foods:

Almonds

Apples

Apricots

Artichokes

Asparagus

Avocados

Beans

Beets

Blackberries

Blackcurrants

Blueberries

Broccoli

Brussels Sprouts

Cabbage

Cantaloupe

Carrots

Cauliflower

Celery

Cherries

Collards

Cucumbers

Fish

Flax/Flaxseeds

Garlic

Grapefruit

Grapes

Green Tea

Kale

Kiwi

Lemons/Limes

Lentils

Mushrooms

Oats

Olive Oil

Onions

Oranges

Papaya

Pears

Peas

Pineapple

Pomegranate

Pumpkin/Pumpkin Seeds

Raspberries

Spinach

Squash

Strawberries

Sunflower Seeds

Sweet Potatoes

Swiss Chard

Turnips (especially greens)

Walnuts

Yogurt

Foods To Avoid:

Alcohol

Dairy Products

Eggplant

Eggs

Food Additives

Fried Foods

Meat (especially red meat)

Potatoes

Processed Foods

Salt

Sugar

Tomatoes

White Rice

Helpful Herbs & Spices:

Alfalfa

Aloe Vera

Basil

Cayenne Pepper

Chili Pepper

Cinnamon

Cloves

Echinacea

Garlic

Ginger

Goldenseal

Horsetail

Licorice

Peppermint

Rosemary

Slippery Elm

Turmeric

Yucca

Vitamins & Minerals:

A, C, D, E, F, Calcium, CoQ10, Folic Acid, Selenium, Zinc

"Disease is the warning, and therefore the friend - not the enemy - of mankind."

— Dr. George S. Weger

Influenza

Healing Foods:

Apple Cider Vinegar

Apples (apple juice)

Bananas

Blackcurrants

Broccoli

Brown Rice

Buckwheat

Cabbage

Carrots

Celery

Coconut

Collards

Cranberries (cranberry juice)

Fish

Grapefruit (grapefruit juice)

Green Tea

Honey

Kale

Lemons/Limes

Mushrooms

Oats

Onions

Oranges (orange juice)

Peppers (Sweet)

Persimmons

Pumpkin Seeds

Raisins

Strawberries

Sweet Potatoes

Tomatoes

Vegetable Juices

Warm Broth

Watercress

Watermelon

Foods To Avoid:

Caffeine

Dairy

Fried Foods

Meat

Processed Foods

Salt

Spicy Foods

Sugar

Helpful Herbs & Spices:

Basil
Cayenne Pepper
Chili Pepper
Cloves
Dandelion
Echinacea

Garlic
Ginger (also ginger ale)
Kelp
Peppermint
Red Clover
Slippery Elm

Vitamins & Minerals:

A, B6, B12, C, D, E, P, Calcium, Pantothenic Acid, Selenium,
Zinc

Insomnia

Healing Foods:

Apple Cider Vinegar

Avocados

Bananas

Beets

Blackcurrants

Brown Rice

Cabbage

Carrots

Celery

Cherries

Collards

Corn

Cucumbers

Dairy Products

Dates

Eggs

Fish

Honey

Kale

Lemons/Limes

Lentils

Low-fat Dairy

Mushrooms

Oats

Potatoes

Poultry (especially turkey)

Pumpkin/Pumpkin Seeds

Sesame Seeds

Spinach

Squash

Strawberries

Sunflower Seeds

Turnips (especially turnip greens)

Yogurt

Foods To Avoid:

Beans

Caffeine

Chili Peppers

Chocolate

Fried Foods

Garlic

Meat

Onions

Spicy Foods   Tomatoes
Sugar

Helpful Herbs & Spices:

Chamomile   Peppermint
Dandelion   Red Clover
Ginger   Tarragon
Hops   Valerian
Passion Flower

Vitamins & Minerals:

B6, B12, D, E, Calcium, Folic Acid, Magnesium, Niacin, Pantothenic Acid, Potassium, Thiamine

"I find medicine is the best of all trades because whether you do any good or not you still get your money."

— (Moliere: "A Physician in Spite of Himself," 1664)

Irritable Bowel Syndrome

Healing Foods:

Apples
Apricots
Artichokes
Asparagus
Avocados
Beets (especially beet greens)
Blackberries
Blueberries
Brown Rice
Cantaloupe
Carrots
Celery
Cherries
Collards
Dates
Figs
Fish
Flax/Flaxseeds
Kale
Kiwi

Lentils
Mushrooms
Okra
Olive Oil
Papaya
Pineapple
Prunes
Pumpkin/Pumpkin Seeds
Raspberries
Spinach
Squash
Strawberries
Sunflower Seeds
Sweet Potatoes
Swiss Chard
Turnips (especially turnip greens)
Watercress
Watermelon
Yogurt

Foods To Avoid:

Alcohol
Artificial Sweeteners

Beans
Broccoli

Cabbage

Caffeine

Cauliflower

Chocolate

Corn

Dairy Products

Eggplant

Eggs

Fried Foods

Grapefruit

High-fat Dairy

Lemons/Limes

Nuts

Oats

Onions

Oranges

Peppers (Sweet)

Potatoes

Raisins

Salt

Spicy Foods

Sugar

Tomatoes

Wheat Germ

Helpful Herbs & Spices:

Alfalfa

Aloe Vera

Cayenne

Chamomile

Cinnamon

Dandelion

Ginger

Milk Thistle

Peppermint

Slippery Elm

Vitamins & Minerals:

A, B3, B5, B6, C, D, E, K, Calcium

Kidneys

Healing Foods:

Apple Cider Vinegar
Apples
Artichokes
Asparagus
Blackberries
Blackcurrants
Blueberries
Broccoli
Brown Rice
Brussels Sprouts
Buckwheat Germ
Cabbage
Carrots
Cauliflower
Celery
Cherries
Coconut
Corn
Cranberries
Cucumbers
Eggplant
Flax/Flaxseeds

Grapefruit
Grapes
Green Tea
Kale
Mango
Mushrooms
Nuts
Okra
Olive Oil
Onions
Peaches
Pears
Peas
Peppers (Sweet)
Pineapple
Raspberries
Squash
Strawberries
Turnips
Walnuts
Watercress
Watermelon

Foods To Avoid:

Apricots
Avocados
Baking Soda
Bananas
Beans
Beets
Carbonated Beverages
Chocolate
Dairy Products
Eggs
Fried Foods
Kiwi
Meat (especially red meat)

Oranges
Potatoes
Processed Foods
Processed Meat
    (including smoked meats)
Prunes
Pumpkin
Raisins
Salt
Spinach (cooked)
Sugar
Sweet Potatoes
Tomatoes

Helpful Herbs & Spices:

Alfalfa
Cayenne Pepper
Chamomile
Cloves
Dandelion
Garlic

Ginkgo Biloba
Horsetail
Kelp
Red Clover
Uva Ursi

Vitamins & Minerals:

B1, B2, B6, B12, C, D, Biotin, Calcium, Folic Acid, Iron, Niacin, Pantothenic Acid, Potassium

Liver

Healing Foods:

Apples

Artichokes

Asparagus

Avocados

Beans

Beets

Blackberries

Blackcurrants

Blueberries

Broccoli

Brown Rice

Brussels Sprouts

Buckwheat Germ

Cabbage

Carrots

Cauliflower

Cherries

Coconut

Collards

Cranberries

Fish

Flax/Flaxseeds

Grapefruit

Green Tea

Honey

Kale

Lemons/Limes

Mango

Okra

Olive Oil

Onions

Oranges

Papaya

Peaches

Peas

Peppers (Sweet)

Raspberries

Sesame Seeds

Spinach

Squash

Strawberries

Sweet Potatoes

Tomatoes

Turmeric

Turnips (especially turnip greens)

Wheat Germ

Yogurt

Foods To Avoid:

Alcohol

Artificial Sweeteners

Dairy Foods

Fried Foods

Meat

Nuts

Processed Foods

Processed Meat (including smoked meat)

Salt

Sugar

White Flour

Helpful Herbs & Spices:

Alfalfa

Aloe Vera

Basil

Cardamom

Cayenne Pepper

Chamomile

Cloves

Dandelion

Echinacea

Ginger

Hops

Licorice

Milk Thistle

Peppermint

Rosemary

Tarragon

Uva Ursi

Vitamins & Minerals:

A, B2, C, D, E, Calcium, Folic Acid, L-Carnitine, Magnesium, Pantothenic Acid, Zinc

Lungs

Healing Foods:

Almonds

Apples

Asparagus

Avocados

Bananas

Beans

Blueberries

Broccoli

Brown Rice

Brussels Sprouts

Buckwheat Germ

Cabbage

Cantaloupe

Carrots

Cauliflower

Collards

Corn

Cranberries

Dates

Eggs

Figs

Fish

Flax/Flax Seeds

Garlic

Grapes

Green Tea

Honey

Kale

Mango

Mushrooms

Oats

Onions

Oranges

Papaya

Peaches

Pears

Peas

Peppers (Sweet)

Persimmon

Pineapple

Pumpkin/Pumpkin Seeds

Spinach

Squash

Strawberries

Sweet Potatoes

Swiss Chard

Tomatoes   Watercress

Turnips   Watermelon

Walnuts

Foods To Avoid:

Alcohol   High-fat Dairy

Caffeine   Meat (especially red meat)

Carbonated Beverages   Processed Meat (including
                                    smoked meat)
Chocolate
                                Salt
Dairy
                                Sugar
Fried Foods

Helpful Herbs & Spices:

Alfalfa   Kelp

Aloe Vera   Licorice

Cardamom   Red Clover

Cayenne Pepper   Rosemary

Garlic   Slippery Elm

Ginger   St. Johns Wort

Goldenseal   Turmeric

Horsetail

Vitamins & Minerals:

A, C, D, E, Folate, Magnesium

"The basic conditions which lead to disease are either nutrient deficiencies or toxic accumulations in the body."

— Dr. Bernard Jensen

Lupus

Healing Foods:

Apricots	Oats
Asparagus	Olive Oil
Avocados	Oranges
Bananas	Peas
Blackberries	Pineapple
Blueberries	Pomegranate
Broccoli	Pumpkin/Pumpkin Seeds
Brown Rice	Raspberries
Brussels Sprouts	Sesame Seeds
Cabbage	Spinach
Cantaloupe	Squash
Eggs	Strawberries
Fish	Sweet Potatoes
Flax/Flaxseed	Swiss Chard
Kale	Yogurt
Low-fat Dairy	

Foods To Avoid:

Beans	Eggplant
Caffeine	Food Additives (especially MSG)
Carbonated Beverages	High-fat Dairy
Cinnamon	Lentils
Corn	

Licorice

Meat (especially red meat and processed meats)

Mushrooms (uncooked)

Nuts

Peppers (Sweet)

Potatoes

Processed Foods

Salt

Soy

Spicy Foods

Sugar

Tomatoes

Wheat

Helpful Herbs & Spices:

Alfalfa

Aloe Vera

Bee Pollen

Cloves

Garlic

Goldenseal

Milk Thistle

Red Clover

Vitamins & Minerals:

A, B6, B12, C, D, E, Calcium, CoQ10, Magnesium, Selenium, Zinc

Menopause

Healing Foods:

Apples	Lemons/Limes
Asparagus	Low-fat Dairy
Avocados	Olive Oil
Bananas	Onions
Beans	Oranges
Beets	Pears
Blueberries	Peas
Broccoli	Peppers (Sweet)
Brown Rice	Prunes
Cabbage	Raspberries
Cantaloupe	Spinach
Carrots	Squash
Cauliflower	Strawberries
Collards	Sweet Potatoes
Cucumbers	Swiss Chard
Eggs	Tomatoes
Fish	Turnips
Flax/Flaxseeds	Walnuts
Grapefruit	Wheat Germ
Grapes	Yogurt
Kale	

Foods To Avoid:

Caffeine

Carbonated Beverages

High-fat Dairy

Processed Foods

Processed Meat

Red Meat

Salt

Spicy Foods

Sugar

Helpful Herbs & Spices:

Aloe Vera

Cinnamon

Dandelion

Gotu Kola

Hops

Kelp

Licorice

Milk Thistle

Passion Flower

Pomegranate

Sage

St. Johns Wort

Sweet Potatoes

Tarragon

Uva Ursi

Valerian

Vitamins & Minerals:

A, B3, B5, B6, B12, C, D, E, Calcium, Iron, Magnesium, Pantothenic Acid

Multiple Sclerosis

Healing Foods:

Apples	Eggs
Apricots	Figs
Asparagus	Fish
Avocados	Flax/Flaxseeds
Bananas	Grapefruit
Beans	Green Tea
Beets	Kale
Blackberries	Kiwi
Blackcurrants	Lemons/Limes
Blueberries	Lentils
Brazil Nuts	Mango
Broccoli	Mushrooms
Brown Rice	Nuts (lactic acid foods)
Brussels Sprouts	Oats
Buckwheat Germ	Olive Oil
Cabbage	Onions
Cantaloupe	Oranges
Carrots	Papaya
Cauliflower	Peaches
Cherries	Peas
Collards	Peppers (Sweet)
Dairy Products	Persimmons
Dates	Pineapple

Potatoes

Pumpkin/Pumpkin Seeds

Raisins

Spinach

Squash

Strawberries

Sunflower Seeds

Sweet Potatoes

Swiss Chard

Tomatoes

Turnips

Walnuts

Watercress

Yogurt

Foods To Avoid:

Alcohol

Caffeine

Chocolate

Cinnamon

Corn

Dairy

Food Additives
(and preservatives)

Fried Foods

Meat (including processed and
smoked meat)

Processed Foods

Salt

Sugar

Wheat

White Flour

Helpful Herbs & Spices:

Alfalfa

Cloves

Dandelion

Garlic

Ginkgo Biloba

Goldenseal

Kelp

Milk Thistle

Oil

Red Clover

Turmeric

Vitamins:

A, B1, B2, B6, B12, C, E, Calcium, CoQ10, Inositol, Isoleucine, L-Lysine, Leucine, Lecithin, Manganese, Magnesium, Selenium, Potassium, Zinc

*"Never, no never does Nature say
one thing and wisdom another."*

— Johann Christolph Frederick von Schuller

Muscles/Ligaments

Healing Foods:

Almonds

Apples

Asparagus

Avocados

Beans

Beets

Blackberries

Blackcurrants

Blueberries

Brazil Nuts

Broccoli

Brussels Sprouts

Cabbage

Cantaloupe

Carrots

Cauliflower

Celery

Collards

Cucumber

Dates

Figs

Flax/Flaxseeds

Grapes

Green Tea

Kale

Lemons/Limes

Lentils

Low-fat Dairy

Mango

Mushrooms

Olive Oil

Onions

Peas

Pineapple

Pomegranate

Potatoes

Pumpkin/Pumpkin Seeds

Raspberries

Spinach

Squash

Strawberries

Sunflower Seeds

Swiss Chard

Tomatoes

Turnips

Walnuts

Watercress

Yogurt

Foods To Avoid:

Alcohol (especially beer)
Artificial Sweeteners
Carbonated Beverages
Caffeine
Chocolate
Honey
High-fat Dairy

Meat (especially red meat)
Peppers (Sweet)
Processed Meat
Processed Foods
Salt
Sugar
White Flour

Helpful Herbs & Spices:

Cayenne Pepper
Dandelion
Garlic
Horsetail

Peppermint
Sage
Turmeric

Vitamins & Minerals:

A, B1, B3, B6, B12, C, D, E, Biotin, Calcium, L-Lysine, Magnesium, Potassium, Zinc

Nausea

Healing Foods:

Apples (applesauce)

Apricots (canned)

Bananas

Brown Rice

Cranberries (juice)

Eggs

Grapes

Green Tea

Honey

Lemons/Limes

Low-fat Dairy

Oats (oatmeal)

Oranges

Peaches (canned)

Yogurt (low-fat)

Foods To Avoid:

Caffeine

Fried Foods

High-fat Dairy

Processed Meat (especially smoked)

Spicy Food

Sugar

Helpful Herbs & Spices:

Alfalfa

Basil

Cardamom

Chamomile

Cinnamon

Cloves

Ginger

Kelp

Peppermint

Turmeric

Vitamins & Minerals:

B6, B12, Folic Acid

"I take the ninja approach to weight loss. If you lose a lot of weight quickly it'll gang up and catch back up with you. But if you sneak away slowly, by the time it realizes you're gone it can't find you anymore."

— Unknown

Nervousness

Healing Foods:

Apple Cider Vinegar	Kale
Apples	Lentils
Asparagus	Low-fat Dairy
Avocados	Mushrooms
Bananas	Oats
Beans	Oranges
Beets	Peaches
Blackberries	Peas
Blueberries	Potatoes
Brazil Nuts	Prunes
Broccoli	Raspberries
Brown Rice	Sesame Seeds
Buckwheat	Spinach
Cabbage	Squash
Celery	Strawberries
Collards	Sweet Potatoes
Eggplant	Walnuts
Fish	Wheat Germ
Flax/Flaxseeds	Yogurt
Green Tea	

Foods To Avoid:

Alcohol	Artificial Sweeteners

Caffeine

Carbonated Beverages

High-fat Dairy

Processed Foods (and additives like MSG)

Salt

Sugar

Helpful Herbs & Spices:

Basil

Chamomile

Ginger

Ginkgo Biloba

Goldenseal

Hops

Milk Thistle

Passion Flower

Red Clover

Sage

St. Johns Wort

Tarragon

Valerian

Vitamins & Minerals:

B1, B2, B3, B6, B12, C, E, Calcium, Folic Acid, Iodine, Iron, Magnesium, Selenium, Zinc

Obesity

Healing Foods:

Apple Cider Vinegar

Apples

Apricots

Artichokes

Asparagus

Beans

Beets

Blackberries

Blueberries

Broccoli

Brown Rice

Brussels Sprouts

Buckwheat Germ

Cabbage

Cantaloupe

Carrots

Cauliflower

Celery

Cherries

Collards

Cranberries

Cucumbers

Dates

Eggplant

Eggs

Figs

Fish

Flax/Flaxseeds

Grapes

Green Tea

Honey

Kale

Kiwi

Lemons/Limes

Lentils

Low-fat Dairy

Mango

Mushrooms

Oats

Okra

Onions

Oranges

Papaya

Peaches

Pears

Peas

Peppers (Sweet)

Pineapple

Pomegranate

Pumpkin/Pumpkin Seeds

Raspberries

Sesame Seeds

Spinach

Squash

Strawberries

Sweet Potatoes

Tomatoes

Turnips

Watercress

Watermelon

Wheat Germ

Yogurt

Foods To Avoid:

Artificial Sweeteners

Caffeine

Chocolate

Dried Fruits

Fried Foods

Fruit Juice

High-fat Dairy

High-fat Salad Dressings

Meat

Nuts

Peanut Butter

Processed Meats

Salt

Shortening

Sugar

White Flour

Help ful Herbs & Spices:

Alfalfa

Aloe Vera

Bee Pollen

Cayenne Pepper

Chili Peppers

Cinnamon

Cloves

Curry

Dandelion

Garlic

Ginger

Goldenseal

Gotu Kola

Hawthorn

Hops

Horsetail

Kelp   Turmeric
Red Clover   Uva Ursi

Vitamins & Minerals:

B12, C, D, E, Calcium, Iodine, Lecithin, Magnesium,
Potassium

Osteoporosis

Healing Foods:

Almonds

Bananas

Beans

Beets

Broccoli

Brown Rice

Carrots

Cauliflower

Coconut

Collards

Eggs

Fish

Flax/Flaxseeds

Grapefruit

Grapes

Honey

Kale

Low-fat Dairy

Mushrooms

Oats

Okra

Olive Oil

Onions

Oranges

Pineapple

Prunes

Pumpkin/Pumpkin Seeds

Raisins

Sesame Seeds

Spinach

Squash

Sweet Potatoes

Swiss Chard

Tomatoes

Turnips (especially turnip greens)

Walnuts

Wheat Germ

Yogurt

Foods to avoid:

Alcohol

Caffeine

Carbonated Beverages

Chocolate

High-fat Dairy

Meat (especially red,
    processed, and
    smoked meat)

Salt

Sugar

Helpful Herbs & Spices:

Alfalfa

Dandelion

Garlic

Horsetail

Kelp

Red Clover

Vitamins & Minerals:

C, D, K, Calcium, Iodine, L-Lysine, Magnesium, Potassium, Zinc

Pain

Healing Foods:

Apples
Apricots
Avocados
Bananas
Beans
Beets
Blackberries
Blackcurrants
Blueberries
Broccoli
Buckwheat Germ
Cabbage
Cantaloupe
Carrots
Cauliflower
Celery
Cherries
Cucumbers
Dates
Figs

Fish
Flax/Flaxseeds
Grapes
Kale
Mango
Mushrooms
Papaya
Peaches
Pears
Peppers (Sweet)
Potatoes
Pumpkin Seeds
Raisins
Spinach
Squash
Strawberries
Sweet Potatoes
Swiss Chard
Turnips
Yogurt

Foods To Avoid:

Caffeine
Chocolate

Corn
High-fat Dairy

Lemons/Limes

Meat

Nuts

Salt

Sugar

Helpful Herbs & Spices:

Basil

Chamomile

Chili Pepper

Garlic

Ginger

Peppermint

Turmeric

Valerian

Yucca

Vitamins & Minerals:

B6, C, E, Calcium, Selenium

Pancreas

Healing Foods:

Beans	Kale
Blueberries	Kiwi
Broccoli	Mushrooms
Brown Rice	Oats
Brussels Sprouts	Olive Oil
Cabbage	Onions
Carrots	Oranges
Cauliflower	Pineapple
Celery	Potatoes
Cherries	Raspberries
Coconut	Spinach
Collards	Squash
Grapefruit	Sweet Potatoes
Grapes	Swiss Chard
Green Tea	Yogurt

Foods to Avoid:

Alcohol	Fried Foods
Caffeine	High-fat Dairy
Carbonated Beverages	Peppers (Sweet)
Corn	Processed Foods
Eggplant	Processed Meat
Eggs	Red Meat

Salt
Spicy Foods
Sugar
Tomatoes

Wheat
White Flour
White Rice

Helpful Herbs & Spices:

Cinnamon
Cloves
Dandelion
Echinacea
Garlic
Ginger

Goldenseal
Horsetail
Licorice
Milk Thistle
Red Clover
Uva Ursi

Vitamins & Minerals:

A, B3, B5, B12, C, D, E, CoQ10, Calcium, Iron, Magnesium, Selenium, Zinc

"Thy food shall be thy remedy."

— Hippocrates

Parkinson's Disease

Healing Foods:

Apples

Artichokes

Asparagus

Avocados

Bananas

Beans

Beets

Blackberries

Blueberries

Broccoli

Brown Rice

Cantaloupe

Carrots

Cauliflower

Collards

Cranberries

Eggs

Fish

Flax/Flaxseeds

Grapefruit

Green Tea

Kale

Kiwi

Lentils

Oats

Okra

Papaya

Pears

Peas

Peppers (Sweet)

Potatoes

Raspberries

Sesame Seeds

Spinach

Squash

Strawberries

Sweet Potatoes

Swiss Chard

Tomatoes

Walnuts

Watermelon

Wheat Germ

Yogurt

Foods To Avoid:

Alcohol

Caffeine

Carbonated Beverages

Fried Foods

High Fat Dairy

Processed Foods

Processed Meats (especially smoked meats)

Red Meat

Salt

Spicy Foods

Sugar

Helpful Herbs & Spices:

Cloves

Dandelion

Echinacea

Garlic

Ginkgo Biloba

Hawthorn

Milk Thistle

Passion Flower

Red Clover

Turmeric

Vitamins & Minerals:

A, B6, C, D, E, Calcium, CoQ10, Glutathione, Selenium

Phlegm

Healing Foods:

Apple Cider Vinegar

Asparagus

Beets

Carrots

Cauliflower

Celery

Grapefruit

Honey

Lemons/Limes

Okra

Onions

Oranges

Pineapple

Raspberries

Spinach

Swiss Chard

Tomatoes

Watercress

Watermelon

Foods To Avoid:

Alcohol

Bananas

Beans

Cabbage

Chocolate

Eggs

Fried Foods

Grapes

High-fat Dairy

Meat

Processed Foods

Processed Meat

Salt

Sugar

Wheat Germ

White Flour

Yogurt

Herbs & Spices:

Cayenne Pepper   Licorice
Chili Pepper   Peppermint
Echinacea   Red Clover
Garlic   Rosemary
Ginger   Sage
Goldenseal   Slippery Elm
Horsetail   Uva Ursi

Vitamins & Minerals:

A, B, C, E, Folic Acid

Pneumonia

Healing Foods

At the beginning stages of pneumonia (during high fever), only vegetable juices should be taken. After that the following foods are beneficial:

Apples	Honey
Artichokes	Lemons/Limes
Beans	Oranges
Beets	Pears
Broccoli	Peas
Brussels Sprouts	Peppers (Sweet)
Cantaloupe	Pineapple
Carrots	Potatoes
Celery	Pumpkin Seeds
Collards	Sesame Seeds
Cranberries	Sunflower Seeds
Eggplant	Spinach
Eggs	Sweet Potatoes
Fish	Tomatoes
Grapefruit	Turnips
Green Tea	

Foods To Avoid:

Alcohol	Dairy Products
Caffeine	Fried Foods

Processed Foods   Sugar
Red Meat   Wheat Flour
Rice   White Flour

Herbs/Spices:

Cayenne Pepper   Ginger
Echinacea   Licorice
Garlic   Slippery Elm

Vitamins & Minerals:

A, B6, C, D, E, Calcium, Folic Acid, Magnesium, Potassium, Selenium, Zinc

Premenstrual Syndrome

Healing Foods:

Almonds

Apple Cider Vinegar

Asparagus

Avocados

Bananas

Beans

Beets

Brazil Nuts

Broccoli

Brown Rice

Carrots

Celery

Coconut

Collards

Corn

Cranberries

Cucumbers

Fish

Flax/Flaxseeds

Grapefruit

Kale

Lemons/Limes

Lentils

Low-fat Dairy

Oats

Onions

Oranges

Peas

Peppers (Sweet)

Potatoes

Pumpkin Seeds

Raspberries

Spinach

Squash

Sunflower seeds (unsalted)

Sweet Potatoes

Swiss Chard

Tomatoes

Walnuts

Watercress

Wheat Germ

Yogurt

Foods To Avoid:

Alcohol	Processed Foods
Caffeine	Processed Meats
Fried Foods	Salt
High-fat Dairy	Sugar
Meat	White Flour

Helpful Herbs & Spices:

Cayenne Pepper	Kelp
Chamomile	Licorice
Cinnamon	Milk Thistle
Dandelion	Passion Flower
Garlic	Peppermint
Ginger	Rosemary
Hawthorn	Valerian

Vitamins & Minerals:

A, B6, C, D, E, Calcium, Magnesium

Prostate

Healing Foods:

Apples
Apricots
Asparagus
Beans
Beets
Brazil Nuts
Broccoli
Brown Rice
Cabbage
Carrots
Cauliflower
Eggs
Fish
Flax/Flaxseeds
Grapes
Grapefruit
Green Tea
Kale
Lemons/Limes

Low-fat Dairy
Mushrooms
Onions
Oranges
Papaya
Peppers (Sweet)
Potatoes
Pumpkin Seeds
Raspberries
Spinach
Squash
Strawberries
Sunflower Seeds
Sweet Potatoes
Swiss Chard
Tomatoes
Watermelon
Wheat Germ

Foods To Avoid:

Alcohol
Caffeine

Fried Foods
High-fat Dairy

Meat (including processed meat)

Processed Foods

Spicy Foods

Sugar

White Flour

White Rice

Helpful Herbs & Spices:

Bee Pollen

Cloves

Echinacea

Garlic

Horsetail

Kelp

Milk Thistle

Red Clover

Turmeric

Uva Ursi

Vitamins & Minerals:

A, B6, C, D, E, F, Selenium, Zinc

…*"The doctor of the future will no longer treat the human frame with drugs, but rather will cure and prevent disease with nutrition."*

— Thomas Edison

Rheumatism

Healing Foods:

Apples
Artichokes
Asparagus
Beans
Blueberries
Broccoli
Brown Rice
Brussels Sprouts
Carrots
Celery
Cherries
Collards
Eggs (especially Omega-3 enriched)
Fish
Flax/Flaxseed
Grapefruit

Grapes
Honey
Kale
Kiwi
Lemons/Limes
Lentils
Oranges
Peaches
Pears
Peas
Pineapple
Raspberries
Squash
Strawberries
Sweet Potatoes
Walnuts

Foods To Avoid:

Caffeine
Corn
Dairy Products
Eggplant
Fried Foods

Meat (especially red meat)
Oats
Peppers (Sweet)
Potatoes
Processed Foods

Processed Meats
Salt
Sugar

Tomatoes
Wheat Flour

Helpful Herbs & Spices:

Alfalfa
Cayenne Pepper
Garlic

Ginger
Red Clover
Turmeric

Vitamins:

B6, B12, C, D, E, Calcium, Folic Acid, Magnesium, Potassium, Selenium, Zinc

Rosacea

Healing Foods:

Apples	Grapefruit
Apricots	Grapes
Artichokes	Kale
Asparagus	Kiwi
Beets	Lentils
Blackberries	Mango
Blueberries	Okra
Broccoli	Papaya
Brown Rice	Pears
Brussels Sprouts	Persimmons
Cabbage	Pomegranate
Cantaloupe	Pumpkin
Carrots	Spinach
Cauliflower	Squash
Celery	Sweet Potatoes
Collards	Swiss Chard
Cranberries	Turnips
Cucumber	Watermelon
Flax (not flaxseeds)	

Foods To Avoid:

Alcohol	Black Pepper
Artificial Sweeteners	Caffeine

Carbonated Beverages

Cayenne Pepper

Cherries

Chili Peppers

Chocolate

Cloves

Corn

Curry

Dairy products

Eggplant

Food Additives
   (especially MSG)

Fried Foods

Garlic

Hot Foods and Beverages

Lemons/Limes

Meat (especially red meat)

Mushrooms

Nuts (all kinds)

Onions

Oranges

Peppers (Sweet)

Pineapple

Processed Foods

Raisins

Raspberries

Seeds (all kinds)

Shellfish

Spicy Foods

Strawberries

Sugar

Tomatoes

Vinegar

Helpful Herbs & Spices:

Alfalfa

Aloe Vera

Basil

Chamomile

Dandelion

Ginger

Kelp

Licorice

Milk Thistle

Red Clover

Rosemary

Sage

Turmeric

Vitamins & Minerals:

A, B3, B12, C, E, Zinc

Shingles

Healing Foods:

Apple Cider Vinegar

Apricots

Asparagus

Avocados

Bananas

Beans

Beets (especially greens)

Blackberries

Blueberries

Brazil Nuts

Broccoli

Brown Rice

Brussels Sprouts

Buckwheat Germ

Cabbage

Carrots

Celery

Cranberries

Cucumbers

Dates

Eggs

Fish

Flax/Flaxseeds

Grapefruit

Grapes

Kale

Kiwi

Lemons/Limes

Low-fat Dairy

Mango

Oats

Okra

Onions

Oranges

Peaches

Pears

Pineapple

Potatoes

Pumpkin

Spinach

Squash

Strawberries

Sweet Potatoes

Swiss Chard

Turnips (especially greens)

Watercress

Watermelon

Yogurt

Foods To Avoid:

Alcohol (especially red wine and beer)

Almonds

Caffeine

Carbonated Beverages

Chocolate

Coconut

Corn (especially popcorn)

Eggplant

Fried Foods

Mushrooms

Peas

Sesame Seeds

Sugar

Sunflower Seeds

Tomatoes

Wheat Germ

Helpful Herbs & Spices:

Alfalfa

Aloe Vera

Cayenne Pepper

Chamomile

Chile Peppers

Cloves

Dandelion

Echinacea

Garlic

Ginger

Goldenseal

Licorice

Milk Thistle

Passion Flower

Peppermint

Rosemary

Sage

St. Johns Wort

Vitamins & Minerals:

A, B12, C, D3, E, L-Lysine, Zinc

Sinus

Healing Foods:

Apple Cider Vinegar	Honey
Apples	Kale
Apricots	Lemons/Limes
Artichokes	Mango
Beans	Oranges
Beets	Papaya
Blackberries	Peaches
Blueberries	Pears
Broccoli	Peppers (Sweet)
Brussels Sprouts	Pineapple
Cabbage	Pumpkin/Pumpkin Seeds
Carrots	Raspberries
Celery	Spinach
Fish	Strawberries
Garlic	Tomatoes
Grapefruit	Walnuts
Green Tea	Yogurt

Foods To Avoid:

Alcohol	Dairy Products
Caffeine	Eggs
Carbonated Beverages	Food Additives (especially MSG)
Corn	

Fried Foods   Rice
Meat (especially smoked meat)   Sugar
Oats   Wheat Germ
Potatoes   White Flour
Processed Foods

Helpful Herbs & Spices:

Alfalfa   Garlic
Basil   Ginger
Cardamom   Ginkgo Biloba
Cayenne Pepper   Goldenseal
Chili Pepper   Horsetail
Cloves   Red Clover
Dandelion   Turmeric

Vitamins & Minerals:

A, C, E, Calcium, Zinc

Skin

Healing Foods:

Almonds

Apple Cider Vinegar

Apricots

Avocados

Beets

Blackberries

Blueberries

Brazil Nuts

Cantaloupe

Carrots

Coconut

Fish

Flax/Flaxseeds

Grapes

Green Tea

Kale

Lemons/Limes

Low-fat Dairy

Mango

Oats

Olive Oil

Papaya

Peaches

Peas

Pomegranate

Spinach

Strawberries

Walnuts

Watermelon

Wheat Germ

Yogurt

Foods To Avoid:

Alcohol

Artificial Sweeteners

Caffeine

Carbonated Beverages

Chocolate

Food Additives

Fried Foods

Meat (especially red meat)

Processed Foods

Processed Meat

Salt   White Flour
Spicy Foods   White Rice
Sugar

Helpful Herbs & Spices:

Alfalfa   Goldenseal
Aloe Vera   Horsetail
Cloves   Kelp
Dandelion   Red Clover
Ginger   St. Johns Wort
Ginkgo Biloba   Tarragon

Vitamins & Minerals:

A, B6, C, E, Biotin (vitamin H), Calcium, Iodine, Selenium, Zinc

Stress

Healing Foods:

Almonds

Apricots

Asparagus

Avocados

Bananas

Beans

Blackberries

Blueberries

Brazil Nuts

Broccoli

Brown Rice

Brussels Sprouts

Cabbage

Cantaloupe

Coconut

Collards

Corn

Eggs

Fish

Grapefruit

Kale

Kiwi

Lemons/Limes

Lentils

Low-fat Dairy

Meat (especially red meat)

Oranges

Papaya

Peas

Peppers (Sweet)

Potatoes

Raspberries

Spinach

Strawberries

Sunflower Seeds

Sweet Potatoes

Swiss Chard

Tomatoes

Wheat Germ

Yogurt

Foods To Avoid:

Alcohol

Caffeine

Carbonated Beverages

Chocolate

Food Additives   Processed Meats
High-fat Dairy   Salt
Processed Foods   Sugar

Helpful Herbs & Spices:

Basil   Ginkgo Biloba
Bee Pollen   Hops
Cayenne Pepper   Milk Thistle
Chamomile   Passion Flower
Ginger   Valerian

Vitamins & Minerals:

A, B3, B6, B12, C, E, Calcium, Folic Acid, Iron, Magnesium,
Pantothenic Acid, Potassium, Thiamine, Zinc

Stroke

Healing Foods:

Almonds	Green Tea
Apples	Kale
Apricots	Kiwi
Asparagus	Lemons/Limes
Avocados	Oats
Bananas	Olive Oil
Beans	Oranges
Beets	Peaches
Blackberries	Pears
Blueberries	Peas
Broccoli	Peppers (Sweet)
Brown Rice	Persimmons
Brussels Sprouts	Prunes
Carrots	Spinach
Cauliflower	Strawberries
Cherries	Sunflower Seeds
Collards	Sweet Potatoes
Eggplant	Swiss Chard
Figs	Walnuts
Fish	Watermelon
Flax/Flaxseeds	Wheat Germ
Grapefruit	

Foods To Avoid:

Caffeine   Red Meat
Carbonated Beverages   Salt
High-fat Dairy   Sugar
Processed Foods

Helpful Herbs & Spices:

Chili Pepper   Ginkgo Biloba
Garlic   Gotu Kola
Ginger   Hawthorn

Vitamins & Minerals:

B6, B12, C, Calcium, Folic Acid, Inositol, Magnesium, Niacin, Pantothenic Acid, Potassium, Riboflavin, Thiamine, Zinc

Teeth/Gums

Healing Foods:

Apple Cider Vinegar

Apples

Asparagus

Broccoli

Cabbage

Cantaloupe

Carrots

Cauliflower

Celery

Coconut

Cucumbers

Fish

Green Tea

Kiwi

Low-fat Dairy

Mushrooms

Onions

Oranges

Pears

Peppers (Sweet)

Pineapple

Pomegranate

Sesame Seeds

Spinach

Tomatoes

Turnips

Walnuts

Watermelon

Yogurt

Foods To Avoid:

Bananas

Caffeine

Carbonated Beverages

Dried Fruit

Grapefruit

Honey

Lemons/Limes

Raisins

Sugar

Helpful Herbs & Spices:

Alfalfa   Goldenseal

Aloe Vera   Hawthorn

Cayenne Pepper   Hops

Chamomile   Licorice

Cinnamon   Peppermint

Cloves   Sage

Echinacea   Tarragon

Ginger

Vitamins & Minerals:

A, B2, B12, C, D, E, Calcium, Folic Acid, Iron, Zinc

Thyroid/Goiter

Healing Foods:

Almonds	Oats
Asparagus	Onions
Avocados	Oranges
Bananas	Peas
Beans	Peppers (Sweet)
Blackcurrants	Pineapple
Brazil Nuts	Pumpkin Seeds
Brown Rice	Raisins
Carrots	Raspberries
Cherries	Sesame Seeds
Coconut	Spinach
Dates	Squash
Eggs	Sunflower Seeds
Fish	Sweet Potatoes
Flax/Flaxseeds	Tomatoes
Grapes	Walnuts
Lentils	Watercress
Mango	Watermelon
Mushrooms	Wheat Germ

Foods To Avoid:

Broccoli	Cabbage
Brussels Sprouts	Caffeine

Chocolate   Pears
Corn   Potatoes
Fried Foods   Processed Foods
High-fat Dairy   Salt
Kale   Strawberries
Meat   Sugar
Peaches   White Flour

Helpful Herbs & Spices:

Kelp   Turmeric

Vitamins & Minerals:

A, B1, B2, B3, B6, B12, C, D, E, F, Calcium, Copper,
Manganese, Magnesium, Selenium, Zinc

"The human body heals itself and nutrition provides the resources to accomplish the task."

— Roger Williams Ph.D.

Ulcerative Colitis

Healing Foods:

Apples	Pears (canned)
Avocados	Potatoes (without skin)
Bananas	Raspberries
Blueberries	Squash
Cantaloupe	Strawberries
Fish	Sweet Potatoes
Oranges	Tomatoes
Papaya	Yogurt
Peaches (canned)	

Foods To Avoid:

Alcohol	Chili Pepper
Artificial Sweeteners	Corn (including popcorn)
Beans	Dairy Products
Black Pepper	Dried Fruit
Blackberries	Fried Foods
Blackcurrants	Kale
Brussels Sprouts	Lentils
Cabbage	Meat
Caffeine	Nuts
Carbonated Beverages	Oats
Cauliflower	Pineapple
Cayenne Pepper	Processed Foods

Seeds (all)   Watermelon
Spicy Foods   Wheat Germ
Sugar   White Flour

Helpful Herbs & Spices:

Alfalfa   Ginger
Aloe Vera   Milk Thistle
Chamomile   Red Clover
Cloves   Slippery Elm
Dandelion   Turmeric

Vitamins & Minerals:

A, B6, B12, C, D, E, K, Calcium, Folic Acid, Iron, Magnesium, Potassium, Selenium, Zinc

Ulcers

Healing Foods:

Almonds	Green Tea
Apple Cider Vinegar	Honey
Apples	Kale
Bananas	Oats
Blackberries	Olive Oil
Blackcurrants	Raisins
Blueberries	Raspberries
Buckwheat Germ	Spinach
Celery	Sweet Potatoes
Coconut	Swiss Chard
Cranberries	Yogurt

Foods To Avoid:

Beans	Fried Foods
Broccoli	Garlic
Brussels Sprouts	Grapefruit
Cabbage	Lemons/Limes
Caffeine	Meat (especially red meat)
Carbonated Beverages	Onions
Cauliflower	Oranges
Cayenne Pepper	Peas
Chili Pepper	Peppers (Sweet)
Chocolate	Processed Meats

Spicy Foods	Tomatoes
Sugar	Turnips

Helpful Herbs & Spices:

Alfalfa	Sage
Aloe Vera	Slippery Elm
Ginger	St. Johns Wort
Goldenseal	Turmeric
Hops	Valerian
Horsetail	White Oak Bark
Licorice	Yucca
Passion Flower	

Vitamins & Minerals:

B12, C, E, K, Calcium, Folic Acid, Magnesium, Selenium, Zinc

Urinary Tract

Healing Foods:

Apricots	Green Tea
Asparagus	Lentils
Beans	Oats
Blueberries	Olive Oil
Brazil Nuts	Peppers (Sweet)
Cabbage	Potatoes
Celery	Spinach
Cherries	Squash
Coconut	Sweet Potatoes
Cranberries	Tomatoes
Fish	Yogurt

Foods To Avoid:

Alcohol	Meat (especially red meat)
Caffeine	Oranges
Carbonated Beverages	Processed Foods
Chocolate	Salt
Corn	Spicy Foods
Dairy Products	Sugar
Fried Foods	Wheat Flour
Lemons/Limes	White Flour

Helpful Herbs & Spices:

Cardamom	Milk Thistle
Cats Claw	St. Johns Wort
Echinacea	Turmeric
Horsetail	Uva Ursi

Vitamins & Minerals:

A, B12, C, E, Calcium, Magnesium, Selenium, Zinc

Varicose Veins

Healing Foods:

Apple Cider Vinegar

Apples

Asparagus

Beans

Beets

Blackberries

Blueberries

Broccoli

Buckwheat

Carrots

Cherries

Chocolate (dark)

Collards

Grapefruit

Grapes

Green Tea

Kale

Lemons/Limes

Lentils

Oats

Onions

Oranges

Peppers (Sweet)

Pineapple

Pomegranate

Raspberries

Spinach

Strawberries

Sweet Potatoes

Wheat Germ

Foods To Avoid:

Alcohol

Fried Foods

High Fat Dairy

Meat

Processed Foods

Salt

Sugar

Helpful Herbs & Spices:

Aloe Vera	Ginger
Cayenne Pepper	Ginkgo Biloba
Chamomile	Gotu Kola
Dandelion	Hawthorn
Garlic	

Vitamins & Minerals:

A, B3, B6, B12, C, E, Zinc

...*"Those who think they have no time for healthy eating will sooner or later have to find time for illness."*

— Edward Stanley

Bibliography

Adderly, Brenda D. *The Complete Guide to Nutritional Supplements - Everything You Need To Make Informed Choices for Optimum Health.* Dove Entertainment, 1998.

Balch, James F. MD and Phyllis A Balch, CNC. *Prescription for Nutritional Healing.* New York: Avery Trade, 2008.

Barnard, Neal M.D. *Pain Relief Foods.* Emmaus, Pennsylvania: Rodale Press, 1987.

Berasques, K. "Historical Notes on Rosacea." *European Journal of Dermatology.* 5: pp. 16-22, 1995.

Bingham R, Bellew BA, Bellew JG. "Yucca plant sap in the management of arthritis." J *Appl Nutr* 1975;27:45-50.

Blau, Sheldon Blau and Dodi Schultz. *Living With Lupus, The Complete Guide.* Cambridge, MA: De Capo Press, 2004.

Cabrera C, Artacho R, Gimenez R. "Beneficial effects of green tea--a review." *J Am Coll Nutr.* 2006;25(2):79-99.

Campbell, T. Colin, Ph.D. "The China Study." 2006

Carper, Jean. *Food: Your Miracle Medicine.* New York: Harper Collins, 1993.

Chen, Dr. J. and Dr. J.H. Kang: "Quercetin and trichostatin A cooperatively kill human leukemia cells." *Pharmazie,* Vol 60, No. 11. (November 2005), pp. 856-860

Cousin, Pierre Jean and Kirsten Hartvig. *The Complete Guide To Nutritional Health.* London: Duncan Baird Publishers, 2002.

Covas, MI. "Olive oil and the cardiovascular system." *Pharmacol Res.* Jan 2007.

Cvetnic Z, Vladimir-Knezevic S. "Antimicrobial activity of grapefruit seed and pulp ethanolic extract." *Acta Pharm.* 2004;54(3):243-50.

Das, M, and others. "Inhibition of tumor growth and inflammation by consumption of tea." *Phytother Res.* 2002;16 Suppl 1:S40-4.

Decuypere, Dr. J.D. "Genetically Engineered Foods." *Health Alternatives* 2000.

Dorchies, OM, and others. "Green tea extract and its major polyphenol (-)-epigallocatechin gallate improve muscle function in a mouse model for Duchene muscular dystrophy." *Am J Physiology Cell Physiol.* 2006;290(2):C616-25.

Duke, James A. *Handbook Of Medicinal Herbs.* Boca Raton: CRC Press, 2002.

Faria, D.T., and A. Edward. "Rosacea: Recognition and Management." *Hospital Medicine*, Dec. 1991: pp. 94-106.

Farinotti M, Simi S, Di Pietrantonj C, et al. "Dietary interventions for multiple sclerosis." *Cochrane Database Syst Rev.* 2007;(1):CD004192.

Farooqui AA, Horrocks LA, Farooqui T. "Modulation of inflammation in brain: a matter of fat." *J Neurochem.* 2007 Jan 25.

Foster, S. *101 Medicinal Herbs.* Loveland, CO: Interweave Press, 1998.

Goulart, Frances Sheridan. *Super Healing Foods.* New York: Reward Books, 1995.

Hale, LP and others. "Proteinase activity and stability of natural bromelain preparation." *Int Immunopharmacol.* 2005;5(4):783-93.

Hill, Douglas. *Prevention Natural Healing Guide 2000.* Emmaus, Pennsylvania: Rodale Press, 2000.

Hobbs, Christopher L.Ac. *Natural Therapy for Your Liver.* New York: Avery, 2002.

Hoffman, Jay M. MD. *Hunza, Secrets Of The World's Healthiest And Oldest Living People.* New Win Publishing.

Holtmann G, and others. "Efficacy of artichoke leaf extract in the treatment of patients with functional dyspepsia: a six-week placebo-controlled, double-blind, multicentre trial." *Ailment Pharmacol Ther.* 2003 Dec;18(11-12):1099-105. PMID: 14653829

Hsu TF, Kise M,and others. "Effects of pre-germinated brown rice on blood glucose and lipid levels in free-living patients with impaired fasting glucose or type 2 diabetes.". J Nutr Sci Vitaminol (Tokyo). 2008 Apr;54(2):163-8.

Huang, S.M. and others. "Effects of flavonoids on the expression of the pro-inflammatory response in human monocytes induced by ligation of the receptor for AGEs." *Mol Nutr Food Res.* 2006 Dec;50(12):1129-39.

Huntley, A. "A review of the evidence for efficacy of complementary and alternative medicines in MS." *Int MS J.* 2006 Jan;13(1):5-12, 4.

Jibrin, Janis M.S, R.D. *The Supermarket Diet.* New York: Hearst, 2007.

Johnson SK, Diamond BJ, Rausch S, et al. "The effect of Ginkgo biloba on functional measures in multiple sclerosis: a pilot randomized controlled trial." *Explore (NY)* 2006;2(1):19-24.

Kaikkonen J, Nyyssonen K, Tuomainen TP, et al. "Determinants of plasma coenzyme Q10 in humans." *Federation of European Biochemical Societies Letters* 443(2): 163-166, 1999.

Kan H, Steven J, et al. "Dietary fiber, lung function, and chronic obstructive pulmonary disease in the Atherosclerosis Risk in Communities (ARIC) Study.". American Journal of Epidemiology 2008

Kimball, SM, Ursell MR, O'Connor P, Vieth R. "Safety of vitamin D3 in adults with multiple sclerosis." *J Clin Nutr.* 2007;86(3):645-51.

Kormosh, N, Laktionov K, Antoshechkina M. "Effect of a combination of extract from several plants on cell-mediated and humoral immunity of patients with advanced ovarian cancer." *Phytother Res.* 2006;20(5):424-5.

Kowalchik, Claire & Hylton, William. *Rodale's Illustrated Encyclopedia of Herbs.* Emmanus, Pennsylvania: Rodale Press, 1998.

Kushi, Michio. *Natural Healing through Macrobiotics.* Brookline, Massachusetts: Japan Press, 1978

Lininger, Schuyler W. Jr., D.C.and others. *The Natural Pharmacy - Complete Home Reference to Natural Medicine.* New York: Three Rivers, 1999.

Lyall, K. A. and others. "Short-term blackcurrant extract consumption modulates exercise-induced oxidative stress and lipopolysaccharide-stimulated inflammatory responses." *European Journal of Clinical Nutrition* 56: 1020-1023 2002.

Lopez-Garcia, E, Schulze, M.B. and others. "Major dietary patterns are related to plasma concentrations of markers of inflammation and endothelial dysfunction." *Am J Clin Nutr.* 2004 Oct;80(4):1029-35.

Mark, B.L and J. A. Carson. "Vitamin D and autoimmune disease—implications for practice from the multiple sclerosis literature." *J Am Diet Assoc.* 2006;106(3):418-24.

Matsumoto, H. and others. "Effects of blackcurrant anthocyanin intake on peripheral muscle circulation during typing work in humans." *European Journal of Applied Physiology* 94: 36-45 2005.

McPhee, Stephen J. "Current Medical Diagnosis and Treatment" 2009.

McGuffin M., and others. *American Herbal Products Association's Botanical Safety Handbook.* Boca Raton, Florida: CRC Press, 1997.

McKoewn, L.A. "This Undiagnosed Skin Disease Doesn't Just Go Away." *Medical Tribune Service.* August, 1995.

Mindell, Earl, R.Ph, Ph.D., & Virginia Hopkins. *Prescription Alternatives.* New Canaan: Keats Publishing, 1998.

Mindell Earl, R.Ph.Ph.D. and Carol Coleman. *Earl Mindell's Supplement Bible.* New York: Fireside, 1998.

Moore, M. *Medicinal Plants of the Desert and Canyon West.* Santa Fe: Museum of New Mexico Press, 1989.

Murray, Michael T. ND and Joseph E. Pizzorna, ND. *Encyclopedia of Natural Medicine.* New York: Random House, 1998.

Panush RS, Veloso ML, Weiss S, Bielory L. "Mechanisms in adverse reactions to food. The joints and muscles." *Allergy.* 1995;50(20 Suppl):74-7.

Perricone, Nicholas M.D. *The Perricone Promise.* New York: Warner Books, 2003.

Pitchford, Paul. *Healing With Whole Foods – Asian Traditions and Modern Nutrition.* Berkley: North Atlantic Books, 2002.

Rain, Mary Summer. *Earthway.* New York: Pocket Books, 1990

Robinson, William. "Delay in the Appearance of Palpable Mammary Tumors in C3H Mice Following the ingestion of Pollenized Food." *Journal of the National Cancer Institute,* 1948.

Royal, Penny . *Herbally Yours.* Hurricane, Utah, Sound Nutrition, December, 1976.

Scalzo, Richard & Cruz, Omar. *Traditional Medicines from the Earth.* Brevard , North Carolina: 2007.

Simopoulos AP. "Omega-3 fatty acids in inflammation and autoimmune diseases." *J Am Coll Nutr.* 2002;21(6):495-505.

Thibault, A. and others. "Phase I study of lovastatin, an inhibitor of the mevalonate pathway, in patients with cancer." *Clinical Cancer Research* 2(3): 483-491, 1996.

Thiboutot, D.M. "Acne Rosacea." *American Family Physician.* Dec: pp. 1691-1697, 1994.

Tierra, Michael L.Ac., O.M.D. The Way of Herbs. New York: Pocket Books 1998.

Tourles, Stephanie . *Naturally Healthy Skin.* Pownal, Vermont: Storey Books, 1999

Tyler, Varro E. Ph.D. Sc.D. and others. *The Doctors Book of Herbal Home Remedies - Cure Yourself With Nature's Most Powerful Healing Agents.* Emmaus, Pennsylvania: Rodale 2000.

Watkins BA, Hannon K, Ferruzzi M, Li Y. "Dietary PUFA and flavonoids as deterrents for environmental pollutants." *J Nutr Biochem*. 2007 Mar;18(3):196-205.

Weed, Susun S. and Christiane Northrup. *Breast Cancer, Breast Health! The Wise Woman Way*. Woodstock, New York: Ash Tree Publishing, 1996.

Whitmarsh, T.E. " Homeopathy in multiple sclerosis." *Complement Ther Nurs Midwifery*. 2003;9(1):5-9.

Wilkin, J.K. *"Rosacea: Pathophysiology and Treatment."* Archives of Dermatology. 130: pp. 359-362, 1994.

Wills, Judith. *The Food Bible*. London: Quadrille Publishing, 1998.

Wood, Rebecca. *The New Whole Foods Encyclopedia - Comprehensive Resource for Healthy Eating*. New York: Penguin Books, 1999.

Yian Gu, Ph.D., and others. "Food Combination and Alzheimer's Disease Risk: A Protective Diet." *Archives of Neurology*, Vol. 67(No. 6): April 12, 2010.

Yoon, J.H.and S.J. Baek. "Molecular targets of dietary polyphenols with anti-inflammatory properties." *Yonsei Med J* 2005;46(5):585-96.

Websites

altnature.com: *Gotu Kola* December. 2010

americanchronicle.com: *Coconut Oil: A New Weapon Against AIDS.* Dr. Bruce Fife. February 21, 2009

anti-aging-articles.com: *Olive Oil—An Anti-Aging Food.* December 2010

am-fe.ift.org: *Nutrition Intervention as the Fountain of Youth* Institute of Food Technologists press release June 30, 2008

hsph.harvard.edu/nutritionsource: *Health Gains from Whole Grains.* February 2011

ars.usda.gov: *Can Foods Forestall Aging?* January, 2011

articlesbase.com: *Boost Your Health With Natural Blackberries.* July, 2009.

articlesbase.com: *The Health Benefits of Apricots.* July, 2010.

associatedcontent.com: *The Surprising Health Benefits of Sesame Seeds.* Kristie Leong, M.D., Nov 23, 2010

avocadopoint.com: *Health Benefits of Avocados 2010*

azcentral: *Cinnamon, cloves may spice up health, studies say.* Alan Mozes. April 5, 2006

bees-and-beekeeping.com: *Pollen Extract as Treatment for Enlarged Prostate.* February, 2011

bri.ucla.edu: *Ginkgo Biloba & The Brain: Ginkgo biloba may help improve memory, and could even protect against Alzheimer's.* September, 2006.

calraisins.org: *Raisins' role in the possible prevention of heart disease and certain cancers.* April, 2001

canadacontent.com: *A New Drug—Kiwi.* January, 2011

cancer.gov/cancertopics: *Antioxidents and Cancer Prevention.* January 2011

cancer.org/Healthy/EatHealthyGetActive: *ACS Guidelineson Nutrition Physical Activity for Cancer Prevention:Common Questions About Diet and Cancer.* January 2011

cancer.org: *Echinacea.* Jan 2011

canceractive.com: *Red Clover* February, 2011

cnn.com: *Broccoli beats most other veggies in health benefits.* CNN Health April 17, 2000

corditecountryshownotes.wordpress.com: *The Healing Properties of Winter Squash.* October 2009.

dailymail.co.uk: *Blackcurrants are the berry best fruit for you.* January, 2011

dole.com: Dole Nutrition Institute. *Swiss Chard.* January, 2011

dried-sprouts.com: *Alfalfa Sprouts Improve Cholesterol* Steve Meyerowitz January,2011

drweil.com: *3 Reasons to Eat Turmeric.* January 2011

earthincommon.com: *New Study Finds Kelp Can Reduce Level of Hormone Related to Breast Cancer Risk* January 2011

ehow.com: Natural Foods That Help Depression Selena Templeton January, 2011

en.wikipedia.org 1,2-Dibromo-3-chloropropane March, 2011

ezinearticles.com: *Stay Sharp for Life and Prevent Alzheimer's.* Donna Cope. January 2011

fasting.ws: *Tarragon Cancer Cure.* January 2011

foodnavigator-usa.com: *Potato proteins offer blood pressure benefits.* Stephen Daniells. March 2008

foundhealth.com: *What Is the Scientific Evidence for Valerian?* December 2010

futurity.org: *Watercress may help starve breast cancer.* September 2010.

health.harvard.edu: *Health benefit of pomegranate juice on prostate cancer and the heart.* April 2007

herbcompanion.com: *The Health Benefits of Rosemary.* Jerry Schwartz. January/February 1999 February, 2011

internethealthlibrary.com: *Multiple Sclerosis Research Sunflower Seed Oil and Multiple Sclerosis.* December, 2010

i-sis.org.uk: Institute of Science in Society. *Organic Strawberries Stop cancer Cells.* July 2006

jeunesse-eternelle.com: *Yucca Root.* February 2011

johnshopkinshealthalerts.com: *Gout and Diet.* July 10, 2006

lifemojo.com: *Health Benefits of Tomatoes.* January 13, 2011 lifescript.com: *Carve it Up: Health Benefits of Pumpkin Seeds and More.* Lisa Mosing, MS, RD, FADA. October 2006

livestrong.com: *What are the benefits of garlic in your diet?* January, 2011

livestrong.com: *Milk Thistle's Benefits* January 2011

livestrong.com: *Slippery Elm – a Clean Colon* February, 2011

livestrong.com: *Health Benefits of Cardamom.* January, 2011

livestrong.com: *Milk Thistle Use in Pregnancy.* January 2011

livestrong.com: *Pineapple & Bromelain.* January 2011

livestrong.com: *The Effects of Cayenne Pepper on the Body* Jan 2011

livestrong.com: *What are the benefits of okra for a diabetic patient?* January 2011

livestrong.com: *Benefits of Red Raspberry Tea* January, 2011

livestrong.com: *Benefits of Wheat Germ. January, 2011.*

livestrong.com: *Clear Up Acne* August McLaughlin January, 2011

livestrong.com: *The Best Foods to Prevent Aging* Sarah Davis February, 2011

livestrong.com: *Foods That Cause Alzheimer's Disease* Adam Dave, MD: February, 2011

livestrong.com: *Foods to Eat if Anemic* Laura Candelaria February, 2011

livestrong.com: *Foods That Help Arthritis Sufferers* August McLaughlin February, 2011

livestrong.com: *What Foods Help to Lower Blood Pressure* Jill Corleone February, 2011

livestrong.com: *12 Most Effective Foods for Chronic Bronchitis* August J. McLaughlin February, 2011

livestrong.com *Foods That Fight Cancer* August J. McLaughlin

livestrong.com: *What Foods Should You Avoid When You Have a Cold?* Sarah Dray January, 2011

livestrong.com: *High Fiber Foods That Help Constipation* Sara Irene January, 2011

livestrong.com: *Foods to Avoid with Depression* August J. McLaughlin February, 2011

livestrong.com: *Which Foods Help Treat Depression* August J. McLaughlin February, 2011

livestrong.com: *Foods To Help Diabetes Sugar Levels* Aglaee Jacob February, 2011

livestrong.com: *Foods to Eat or Not to Eat with Diverticulosis* Jill Andrews February, 2011 livestrong.com: *What Foods to Eat to Avoid Gallstones* August J. McLaughlin February, 2011

livestrong.com: *Foods to Help Gas and Bloating* August J. McLaughlin February, 2011

livestrong.com: *Foods that Help with Stress Anxiety* Christine Switzer March, 2011

livestrong.com: *The Best Foods to Eat for Parkinson's Disease* August J. McLaughlin March, 2011

livestrong.com: *Foods That Help a Sinus Infection* Kelly Taylor March, 2011

livestrong.com: *What Foods Help Cure Acne?* August McLaughlin March, 2011

livestrong.com: *Foods That Support Thyroid Function* Geoff Mitchell March, 2011

livestrong.com: *Foods to Eat to Avoid Urninary Tract Infections* Gloria Attar, R.N., B.S.N March, 2011

livestrong.com *Herbs for Radiation Effects* Tracy Planinz March, 2011

lpi.oregonstate.edu: Linus Pauling Institute. *Resveratrol.* 2011

mayoclinic.com: *Aloe Vera.* January 2011

mayoclinic.com: *Ginkgo Biloba.* January 2011

mayoclinic.com: *Prostate cancer prevention: What you can do.* November, 2010

med.umich.edu: *Ginger causes ovarian cancer cells to die, U-M researchers find.* February, 2011

medic8.com: *Black Cohosh and the Symptoms of Menopause.* January 2011.

more.com: *27+ Anti-Aging Superfoods.* February 2008

mskcc.org: *Hops.* February 2011

mypyramid.gov/pyramid/grains: USDA: Inside the Pyramid February 2011

ncbi.nlm.nih.gov: *Preoperative oral Passiflora incarnata reduces anxiety in ambulatory surgery patients: a double-blind, placebo-controlled study.* U.S. National library of Medicine National Institutes of Health June, 2008

ncsweetpotatoes.com: *Sweet Potatoes-Nature's Health Food.* Dr. Robert Cordell. January 2011

nhs.uk/news: *Peppermint does soothe IBS.* November 11, 2008

nih.gov: Stud*ies show chamomile capsules ease anxiety symptoms.* December 2010

npr.org: *Study: Red Rice Yeast Helps Cut Bad Cholesterol.* Allison Aubrey July 1, 2008 nutrigredients-usa.com: Study backs dried for stronger osteoporosis resistance. Stephen Daniells. June 2008.

nutriingredients-usa.com: *Pea protein may cut blood pressure and help kidneys*. Stephen Daniells, March 2009

nutritionandmetabolism.com: *Effects of capsinoid ingestion on energy expenditure and lipid oxidation at rest and during exercise.* Andrea R Josse, and others. *ScienceDaily (Feb. 5, 2001)*

pbs.org The Dirty Dozen and Clean 15 of Produce Jackie Pou March, 2011

qualityhealth.com: *Basil Plants Can Fight Arthritis* By Andrea Neblett. February, 2011

redcrossblood.org: *American Red Cross: Iron Rich Foods* February, 2011

redorbit.com: *International Journal of Obesity Finds Yogurt Promotes Fat Loss.* March, 2005

research.va.gov: *Popular Herb 'Goldenseal' Lowers Cholesterol in Lab Tests* September 21, 2006

science20.com: *Immunological Effect of Active Hexose Correlated Compound (AHCC) in Healthy Volunteers: A Double-Blind, Placebo-Controlled Trial.* Naoyoshi Terakawa, and others. Nutrition and Cancer." January 2009.

sciencedaily.com: *Grapefruit Appears To Lower Cholesterol, Fight Heart Disease.* July 2006. *The Health Benefits of Kale.* Dr. Linda Posh, MS SLP ND. December 2010

sciencedaily.com: *Watermelon Lowers Blood Pressure, Study Finds.* October, 2010.

sciencedaily.com: *Mango Effective in Preventing, Stopping Certain Colon, Breast Cancer Cells, Food Scientists Find.* January 2010.

sciencedaily.com: *Peaches Induce Deliciously Promising Death of Breast Cancer Cells.* June 2010

sciencedaily.com: *A Persimmon A Day Could Be Better For Your Heart Than An Apple.* February 5, 2011

sciencedaily.com: *Mushrooms Could Bolster Your Immune System.* January 2010

squidoo.com: *Lentils Nutritional Information* December, 2010

suite101.com: *The Many Health Benefits of Eating Chillies* Oct 2, 2010 Rachael Ann Loxston

suite101.com: *Can Sage Prevent or Treat Alzheimer's Disease?* Lorena Tonarelli. February, 2011

supplementnews.org: *Uva Ursi Introduction* Feb, 2011

thedietchannel.com: *Do You Have A Nutritional Deficiency? How To Identify The Signs.* Wendy Hodson, ND. January 30, 2007 / *Walnuts slow prostate cancer growth* Janet Raloff. March 27th, 2010

time.com/time/archive: *Foods That Fight Cancer.* Alice Park. April 26, 1999

uconn.edu: *Echinacea Could Cut Chances of Catching Common Cold By More Than Half.* June 26, 2007

umm.edu/altmed/articles: *Acne Overview and Treatment.* December 7, 2008; *Rheumatoid Arthritis,* December 15, 2009;

umm.edu: *Hawthorn.* January 2011

umm.edu: *Dandelion* University of Maryland Medical Center January, 2011

vitaminstuff.com: *Dandelion.* January, 2011.

webmd.com: *Benefits of Flax Seeds.* Elaine Magee, MPH, RD; Louise Chang, MD. November 2010

whfoods.com: *Cantaloupe* Baybutt RC, Hu L, Molteni A. *Vitamin A deficiency injures lung and liver parenchyma and impairs function of rat type II pneumocytes.* May 2000

whfoods.com: *The World's Healthiest Food: Lemons and Limes and Lentils.* January, 2011

whfoods.com: Kritchevsky SB. *Beta-Carotene, carotenoids and the prevention of coronary heart disease.* Journal of Nutrition. January 1999

Magazine Articles, Newspapers, Other Sources

ALZinfo.org.

American Diabetes Association: Carbohydrate Counting

American Heart Association: Potassium and High Blood Pressure

American Institute for Cancer Research: Probiotics for Cancer Prevention?

Arthritis Today: Whole Grains Help You Lose Weight and Fight Inflammation

Chest: *Low Dietary Nutrient Intakes and Respiratory Health in Adolescents*; Jane S. Burns, ScD et al.; May 2007

Cleveland Clinic: Eating for Life: Diet and Diabetes

Cleveland Clinic: Fitting Fiber In

Dental Health Magazine: *Ten Foods for Protecting Your Teeth and Gums.* March 25th, 2008,

Diet.com: Gout Diet

Dr. Northrup: Depression and Dysthmia

Dr. Northrup: Depression and Dysthmia Facts and Treatment Options

Easing Anxiety and Stress Naturally"; Susan M. Lark, M.D.; 1999

Family Doctor: High Blood Pressure: Things You Can Do to Help Lower Yours

Franklin Institute: The Human Brain - Proteins

GiCare: High-Fiber Diet

Gout.com: Understanding Diet

Harvard Health Publications: *Egg Nutrition and Heart Disease. Eggs aren't the dietary demons they're cracked up to be.* July 2006

Herbal Research Publications, February, 2007

Johns Hopkins Medicine: Gout and Diet

Journal of Affective Disorders: *Depression in Parkinson's Disease: A Double-Blind, Randomized, Placebo-Controlled Pilot Study of Omega-3 Fatty-Acid Supplementation;* Ticyana Moralez da Silva et al.; Dec. 2008

Journal of Human Hypertension: *Blood Pressure Response to Calcium Supplementation: A Meta-Analysis of Randomized Controlled Trials*; L.A.J. van Mierlo; 2006

Mayo Clinic.com: High-Fiber Foods

Mayo Clinic: Caffeine and Depression

Mayo Clinic: Gallstones: Alternative Medicine

MayoClinic.com: Alternative Medicine for Dysthymia

MayoClinic.com: Asthma Diet: What You Eat Can Affect Asthma Symptoms

MayoClinic.com: Bloating, Belching and Intestinal Gas

MayoClinic.com: Cold Symptoms: Does Drinking Milk Increase Phlegm?

MayoClinic.com: Colitis: Lifestyle and Home Remedies

MayoClinic.com: DASH Diet: Healthy Eating to Lower Your Blood Pressure

MayoClinic.com: Diabetes Diet: Create Your Healthy-Eating Plan

MayoClinic.com: Diverticulitis Diet

MayoClinic.com: Diverticulitis: Lifestyle and Home Remedies

MayoClinic.com: Diverticulitis: Symptoms

MayoClinic.com: Lifestyle and home remedies

MayoClinic: Gout Diet

Medical News Today: Diet May Help Prevent Allergies and Asthma

MedlinePlus: Antioxidants

MedlinePlus: Gout

Minerva Medica: Female Climacteric Osteoporosis Therapy with Titrated Horsetail (Equisetum Arvense) Extract Plus Calcium (Osteosil Calcium): Randomized Double Blind Study

National Cancer Institute: A Snapshot of Colorectal Cancer

National Cancer Institute: Cancer of the Colon and Rectum: Risk Factors

National Endocrine and Metabolic Diseases Information Service: Hypothyroidism

National Institute of Arthritis and Musculoskeletal and Skin Diseases: Gout

National Institute of Health Office of Dietary Supplements: Iron and Zinc Information

Natural Counselor: Super Unhealthy Foods to Avoid During Cold and Flu Season

NDDIC: Constipation

New England Journal of Medicine

New York-Presbyterian: Want a Healthy Colon? Eat a Rainbow!

Office of Dietary Supplements: Magnesium

Office of Dietary Supplements: Vitamin E Fact Sheet

Overcoming Depression: A Cognitive Therapy Approach Workbook"; Mark Gilson, Arthur Freeman, M. Jane Yates, Sharon Morgillo Freeman; 2009

Practical Kitchen: *Food Combining*. Cheryl Gonzales, RD, CCN 2011

Prevention's Healing with Vitamins"; The Editors of Prevention Health Books.; 1998

St John's Wort for depression (Cochrane Review) abstract Linde K, Mulrow CD, Berner M, Egger M October, 2008

University of Maryland Medical Center: Asthma Facts, Treatment and Lifestyle Suggestions

Robert O. Young D.Sc., Ph.D., *Brussel Sprouts May Prevent or Reverse A Cancerous Condition*. January 13, 2009

Rodale: *Superfish List Reveals Healthiest, Safest Seafood* 2010

SusanMitchell.com: Five Foods to Help Fight a Cold

The Sinus Cure: *7 Simple Steps*; Debra Fulghum Bruce and Murray Grossan; 2007

Tufts University: Omega 3 Fatty Acid Content

U.S. National Library of Medicine: National Institutes of Health: Thyroid

University of Maryland Medical Center *Green Tea* January 2011

University of Maryland Medical Center, Center for Integrative Medicine, Alternative / Complementary Medicine Supplements database.

University of Maryland Medical Center: *Urinary Tract Infection in Women*. December, 2010

University of Maryland Medical Center: Acne

University of Maryland Medical Center: Bronchitis

University of Maryland Medical Center: Bronchitis

University of Maryland Medical Center: Depression Facts and Treatment

University of Maryland Medical Center: Diarrhea

University of Maryland Medical Center: Diverticular Disease

University of Maryland Medical Center: Gallstones and Gallbladder Disease

University of Maryland Medical Center: Hypothyroidism

University of Maryland Medical Center: Irritable Bowel Syndrome Facts and Treatment

University of Maryland Medical Center: Magnesium

University of Maryland Medical Center: Migraines

University of Maryland Medical Center: Omega-3 Fatty Acids

University of Maryland Medical Center: *Osteoporosis.* November, 2010

University of Maryland Medical Center: Parkinson's Disease

University of Maryland Medical Center: Quercetin

University of Maryland Medical Center: Rheumatoid Arthritis

University of Maryland Medical Center: Sinusitis

University of Maryland Medical Center: Ulcerative Colitis -- Treatment

University of Maryland Medical Center: Urinary Tract Infections

University of Michigan Health System: Asthma

University of Michigan Health System: Urinary Tract Infection

University of Michigan Health Systems: Probiotics

University of Sydney: The Glycemic Index

USDA National Nutrient Database: Nutrient Data Laboratory

USDA.gov/Nutrients